This book is a valuable guide for

General Health

Family health

Nutritionists

Health Professionals

Medical Professionals

Biomedical Researchers

&

Biochemists

Unlocking the Mysteries of Nature

Unlock the mysteries of nature by learning to

* heal transient and chronic disorders;

* delay and/or reverse aging;

* generate healthy genes, blood vessels, bones, bone marrow, ligaments and muscles;

* retain clear vision and prevent cataract;

* attain vigor, vitality, a healthy skin tone and youthful appearance;

* achieve a healthy gene expression.

Stay in good health and lead a joyous healthy life!

GROWTH FACTOR:

The Cure for Aging and Chronic Illnesses

SHARWAN KUMAR KAKAR, Ph.D.

VANTAGE PRESS
New York

FIRST EDITION

Copyright © 1996 by Sharwan Kumar Kakar, Ph.D.

Published by Vantage Press, Inc.
516 West 34th Street, New York, New York 10001

Manufactured in the United States of America
ISBN: 0-533-11989-8

Library of Congress Catalog Card No.: 96-90314

0 9 8 7 6 5 4 3 2 1

CHRONIC DISORDERS OF THE HUMAN BODY

Age related disorders: random deterioration or aging hits, decline in organ functions and anatomical modifications.

Bone disorders: abnormalities in bone mass production, arthritis, back pains, metabolic bone diseases, bone infection, osteoporosis and rheumatoid arthritis.

Bone marrow disorders: types of leukemia- lymphogenous and myelogenus.

Carcinogenesis: cancer of bladder, brain, breast, cervix uteri, connective tissue, cranial sinuses, liver, ovary, pancreas, prostate, vagina, mucous membranes and secretive glands.

Gastrointestinal disorders: acidic stomach, peptic ulcer, ulcerative colitis and malabsorption.

General chronic symptoms: anorexia nervosa, chronic fatigue, chronic infection, chronic inflmmation.

Immune system disorders: AIDS, leprosy, T.B., viral hypersensitivity and autoimmune syndrome.

Metabolic disorders: hyper and hypoglycemia, hypo and hyperinsulinism, hyperparathyroidism, hypercalcemia, hypoalbuminemia and hyperlipidemia, dysfunction of endocrine secretion such as hormone.

Nervous system: depression, nervousness, phobia, multiple sclerosis, cerebral atrophy, paralysis, Alzheimer's disease and erosion of epithelial linings in the brain.

Respiratory disorders: common cold, chronic bronchitis, hay fever and sinusitis.

Skin disorders: chronic itching, fungal infection, parakeratosis, psoriasis and skin cancers.

Contents

Prefatory Statement

Every human life ends in death. Most of us have to face the dilemma of old age. Some of us wither gracefully while the others have to go through excruciating pain and suffering before they reach the final destination. The question being raised is: Can an old debilitated body be rejuvenated? In other words, can the quality of life be elevated in old age? Surprisingly, the answer to this ambiguous question is available in this book. This book is unique in many respects because it explains aging, pathogenesis and healing on a scientific basis.

This manuscript represents the summation of several decades of author's original experimental research work with degenerative and chronic disorders of the human body. Based on his experimental results, the author has developed new theories and models to help his readers understand the significance of factors involved in aging and developing chronic disorders. Some of the complex mathematical equations have been avoided to make this book simple and easy to comprehend. This book is both for laymen and professionals who have been searching for answers to such complex issues as life, growth, continuity, disease, old age and death.

ACKNOWLEDGMENTS

The author extends his heartfelt appreciation to Professor Dr. Frederick A. Bettelheim, Ex-chairman, Chemistry Department, for giving him an opportunity to explore literature and research references in biochemical literature, during his stay as a Research Fellow, at Adelphi University, Garden City, N.Y.. He is thankful to Professor Dr. Edward Shenal, Chairman, Chemistry Department, Nassau Community College, Garden City., N.Y., for his moral support. He is grateful to Professor Dr. Joseph Ursino for his participation in discussions about many topics in this book. He expresses his deep appreciation and gratitude to Professor Yeshwant K. Purandare, Ph.D., M.D., Chairman, Chemistry Department, S.U.N.Y., College of Technology, Farmingdale, L.I., N.Y., for reviewing this book and for his helpful suggestions.

Involvement of Central Nervous System in Chronic Diseases

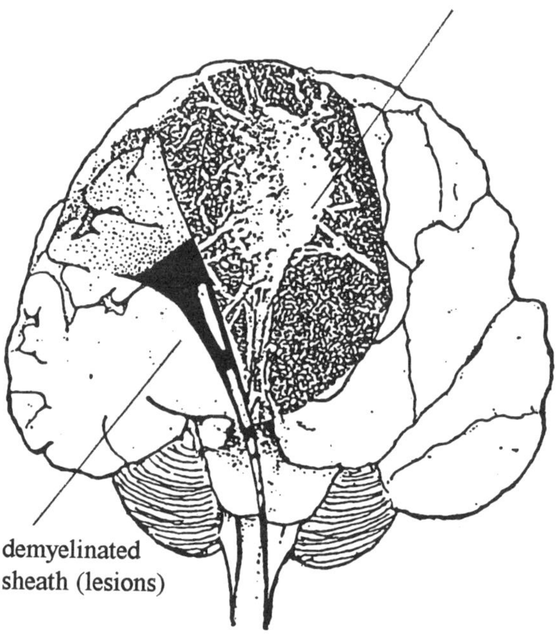

nerve cell

demyelinated
sheath (lesions)

PLATE -I: The right side of the diagram shows the nerve
cell and the left side illustrates the loss of fatty
myelin sheath. Disorders such as Alzheimer's
disease, cerebral atrophy, cerebral palsy,
dementia, encephalomyelitis, multiple sclerosis,
paralysis, retinopathy, etc., are caused by lesions
in myelin sheath.

1 Introduction to Aging

Aging is associated with slow deterioration and oxidation processes.
(Kakar)

Aging is defined as the process of growing old with the passage of time. Why we age is a question the human race has been pondering over for a very long time. To prolong life has been the pursuit of almost all the philosophers of every past civilization. Gerontology - a branch of science that is concerned with the process of growing old (specially among human beings) - has pursued not only the prolongation of life but the prevention and cure of bodily dysfunctions and/or diseases that come with aging.

While it may be so that aging is not necessarily an illness, to some individuals aging involves diminished bodily functions and thus results in illness. Clearly though to some aging can come without having to go through diminished bodily functions which are manifested in marked morphological changes of the anatomy such as a loss in weight, height, and subcutaneous fat from many parts of the body that results in loosening and wrinkling of the skin. There is also the more serious change in the anatomy - the collapse of the vertebrae.

The process of aging may start the day an individual is born or even earlier as some unborn fetus has shown, but the symptoms become more pronounced during the individual's twentieth year and more or less accelerated when the body is in its forty something years. The classical symptoms of aging are well established sooner or later.

Aging of the human body as a whole is an inadequately understood phenomenon. Innumerable views have been advanced, some conflicting and some mutually supporting, but none of them can explain all the facts about the processes involved. The suggestion is often made that aging results from random events termed as aging hits which cause alteration in genes. Another popular view holds that aging results from deterioration because of gene exhaustion. Then there is also the theory that defines aging as deterioration due to free radical mechanism. Surprisingly, there is no general accepted hypothesis that explains all the facts and a great deal of work is needed to substantiate these claims.

From a chemical point of view, aging is associated with slow deterioration and oxidation processes. The changes that take place in an aging body, have indeed very striking similarities with those that are generally noticed in the aging of polymeric materials. The loss of elasticity and flexibility in ligaments, articular cartilage, joint capsules and many bony tissues show with age.

Bones become thin and brittle, they fracture easily with slight physical trauma. This kind of situation is seen in some individuals who suffer from osteoporosis. The fracture of femur caused by a fall, is the most common manifestation. In a more advanced stage of osteoporosis, the body may develop shortening of stature and limitation of physical movements. Other processes such as generation of free radical units, peroxy radical units formation, cross linking , cyclization and hydrogen extraction have been observed in many biologic macromolecules. The other most obvious age related developments are listed below,

*   decrease in adaptability to the environment;
*   decrease in response to specific stimuli;

* decrease in the induction of reductases, hydrolases and lyases but an increase in the induction of transferases;
* loss of microscopic and macroscopic collagen which results in the loss of cell density of many organs and organ systems;
* loss of fatty materials from the central nervous system and thus degenerate the tissues;
* increase in carbohydrates or glucose intolerance which can possibly develop the onset diabetes;
* decline in hepatic and renal functions;
* development of cancers of epithelial and mucosal linings; and
* development of dysfunctional gastrointestinal tract.

Why these changes develop and how they develop will be discussed in this book. But before doing so it might be quite practical to review some of the fundamentals relating to the living body used in the succeeding chapters of interrelating subject matters.

Terms

Morphological changes	*Gerontology*
Subcutaneous fat	*Random events*
Gene exhaustion	*Free radical*
Polymeric material	*Ligaments*
Articular cartilage	*Joint capsule*
Osteoporosis	*Femur*
Peroxy radical	*Crosslinking*
Reductases	*Lyases*
Transferases	*Collagen*
Epithelial and mucosal lining	*Gastrointestinal tract*

2   Building Blocks of Life

Cell is a precise and delicate machinery. Cell for its survival needs nutrients, oxygen and water.

The planet earth is a self contained system. As such very little matter is lost to the outer space. Elements such as hydrogen, carbon, nitrogen, oxygen, phosphorus and sulfur are recycled over and over again to produce a new generation of plants and animals. The earth biosphere is constantly bombarded by solar radiation which play a crucial role in the process of photosynthesis that make life possible. The atmosphere we live in, contains 78% nitrogen, and 21 % oxygen. The remaining gases such as carbon dioxide, noble gases and water vapors make up the rest. Three fourths of our planet is covered with water. It is the main constituent of most living organisms. Many of these organisms live in the ponds, lakes, rivers and the sea. Water is also the major environmental factor that affects our daily life. It is a solvent that dissolves inorganic and organic ions and polar molecules. Most importantly, water is an excellent media for electron transfer which makes possible the many reduction-oxidation mechanisms that form the basis of life.

Oxygen like water is vital to life. It is needed as the final electron acceptor in the process of biochemical oxidation by which cells obtain energy for life processes. On the other hand, the presence of 21 % oxygen is quite high for human purposes and can rapidly oxidize cell components which can be quite dangerous. Therefore, as nature would have it, larger

4

animals including humans, have evolved with specialized respiratory structures that permit them to inhale oxygen in small quantities from the environment and give off carbon dioxide during cellular respiration.

The precursors of living organisms such as amino acids and nucleic acids were originally manufactured by the process of photolysis. The unique combination of these molecules with fats and glucose gave rise to the development of an entity enclosed in a delicate membrane called cell. With the passage of time, diverse types of cells evolved with complex chemistry and chemical structures. Soon multicelluar organisms including man, appeared. Even though the human cell is far more complex than the cells of other organisms, striking similarities exist between them. For instance, cells from both these sources contain approximately, 75-80% water, 12-15 % proteins, 5% fats, 2 % nucleic acids and the remaining are carbohydrates and other substances.

Nucleic acid macromolecules are present in the nucleus of every cell in free as well as in combined form. They are supra large complex molecules. Deoxyribonucleic acid (DNA)- the genetic material- contains instruction for the sequence of amino acids but needs the help of ribonucleic acid (RNA) which takes part in protein synthesis.

In the human body there is an astronomical number of cells and each and every cell contains an exact copy of chromosomes. One can easily realize the importance of DNA constituents needed to make new generation of genes and to replace the damaged or mutated segments in the cells. All these materials come from food.

Proteins form the most abundant component of a cell. They carry out various functions, they act as enzymes to perform

5

many specific biochemical reactions and serve as the structural components for almost all organs of the body. Protein deficiency develops when cells do not receive enough dietary proteins for these functions. The chief source of dietary proteins are meat, milk, poultry, sea food and vegetables.

Fats or lipids constitute 30-40% of total organic matter. The most important lipids are phospholipids. They are similar to triglycerides except that one of the fatty groups is replaced by phosphate and choline residues. Triglycerides that are solid at room temperature are called saturated fats whereas those that are liquid at room temperature are termed as oils. Waxes are esters that are formed from fatty acids and alcohols- chief among them is bees wax.

Carbohydrates play diverse roles in the biological world. The most familiar are sugars, starch and cellulose. Glucose is the most abundant sugar in the world. When many glucose molecules are joined together with the elimination of water, they result in the formation of carbohydrates such as dextrin, glycogen, starch and cellulose. Starches such as corn, potatoes, rice and wheat make up the largest proportion of carbohydrates in the human diet. The body utilizes various types of enzymes to digest and store carbohydrates to derive energy for its maintenance.

The Cell

One of the characteristics of living things is that they have a definite and precise kind of controlled growth mechanism. This is achieved through a highly organized package or fertilized cell which is passed on from generation to generation

6

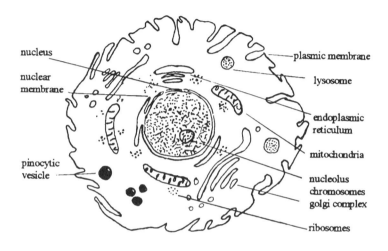

nucleus

nuclear
membrane

pinocytic
vesicle

plasmic membrane

lysosome

endoplasmic
reticulum

mitochondria

nucleolus
chromosomes
golgi complex

ribosomes

Figure 2-1:   General diagram of the cell

to keep the endless rhythm of life. Cell is the smallest building unit of a multicellular organism. The cells of a multicellular organism vary in size and structure. They are conditioned by their adaptation to specific roles in different tissues and organs. Every cell is composed of three principal constituents: plasmic membrane, cytoplasm and the nucleus (Figure 2-1). The plasmic membrane creates a barrier between the external and internal environment. Its primary function is to monitor what enters in and/or leaves the cell. Biological membranes are composed of phospholipids and proteins. Phospholipids form bi-layer in water where the hydrophilic chains are drawn outward and the hydrophobic chains are drawn inward.

Cytoplasm contains subcomponents called organelles such as endoplasmic reticulum, golgi complex, mitochondria, ribosomes and cytoskeletal bodies. Mitochondria are the primary source for generating energy in the cell. They are oval shaped and have cucumber like appearance. One of the structural material called matrix contains most of the enzymes of Krebs cycle. Mitochondria have their own unit of operation for protein synthesis and have the ability to reproduce themselves so that during cell division each cell gets mitochondria. The nucleus is called the brain of the cell and is separated by a double walled membrane termed nuclear membrane. It contains most of the genetic material called DNA and is complexed with basic proteins in a diffused structure called chromatin. It is the function of DNA to transfer hereditary information from one cell to the other and has the instructions for specific protein synthesis coded in its molecular structure. Deoxyribonucleic acid macromolecules do not take part in direct assembly of a protein molecule. The protein synthesis takes place in the cytoplasm. The transfer of instructions from DNA to the site of protein synthesis is carried out by messenger ribonucleic acid (m-RNA). This process of transferring instructions is known as transcription.

8

The message in m-RNA is then utilized to direct the assembly of proper amino acids to synthesize a specific protein. This process is known as translation which is achieved by another type of RNA called transfer RNA (t-RNA). The main purpose of t-RNA is to serve as a carrier for amino acids and also as an interpreter of the genetic code.

The development of a higher organism from a single fertilized egg cell involves a series of steps such as cell growth, cell replication and cell differentiation. The basic characteristic of most of the cells is to divide and reproduce themselves. Besides cell division and cell multiplication, there are other events that are taking place such as change in configuration and function. Cell differentiation is defined as a process by which identical cells acquire different functions such as a muscle cell that contracts. When these differentiated cells are grouped together they form tissues. Further organization of tissues of different types leads to the formation of an organ. Cells carry out many functions in the body and one of those is to make proteins. Cell that does not make proteins is destined for death.

Terms

Photosynthesis	*Biosynthesis*	*Photolysis*
Membrane	*Nucleic acid*	*DNA*
Nucleic acid	*Genetic code*	*m-RNA*
Plasmic membrane	*Cell growth*	*Ribosome*
Golgi complex	*Mitochondria*	*t-RNA*
Cytoskeletal bodies	*Fertilized egg*	*Cell division*
Cell differentiation	*Genetic code*	*Fertilized egg*
Cell replication	*Cell multiplication*	*Transcription*
Plasmic membrane	*Endoplasmic reticulum*	

3   What is Disease?

Diseases acute or chronic are oxidative in nature.
Bacterial and viral attacks in reality are violent oxidative bursts.

What is disease? The word says exactly what it means. Dis-ease or not at ease. When a person is injured by any stimulus, the response to that injury may be manifested by a variety of symptoms such as discomfort and pain. It is this specific language that the body uses to alert the individual to take effective measures to remedy the situation. If the warnings are ignored, the discomfort and pain persist and if allowed to do so, more serious consequences can occur. The process of deterioration may start and in extreme cases result in death. Health, which is the antonym of disease, can be defined as the state of harmony between the internal and external environment.

Diseases can be congenital, inherited, degenerative, infectious or toxin induced. Degenerative diseases include allergic, autoimmune, molecular, metabolic, neoplastic and psychosomatic. The diseases caused inadvertently or otherwise by medical prescription/procedures, is termed as iatrogenic. As described earlier, a disease becomes apparent when there is an alteration in bodily functions and its structural components. Injury to the body can take place at any level: cellular, subcellular, macromolecular or molecular. Cells become diseased due to several reasons. There may be structural changes in the organelles such as membranes, mitochondria or lysosomes. In many cases they

10

may not exhibit any alteration at all and their dysfunctionality may simply be due to lack of specific nutrients. It is important to mention that injury to any cell, tissue or organ can be reversible up to a certain point beyond which there is a point of no return. Necrosis signifies the death of a group of cells caused by an injurious stimulus. The common agents that are capable of inflicting injury, are chemical agents, stress, radiation, extreme temperatures, pressure, bacteria, viruses, fungi and protozoa.

Radiation like infrared, UV, X-rays, γ-rays and high energy ionizing particles can cause dissociation of chemical bonds of chromosomes, lipids and proteins leading to the generation of free radical units. In the absence of oxygen, these radical units tend to stabilize by various mechanisms such as hydrogen transfer, chain extension, cyclization and crosslinking. In the presence of oxygen peroxy radical units are formed, which after stabilization leads to the formation of epoxy, hydroxy and carboxylic acid derivatives. Peroxy radical units generate heat in the body. Dissociation and free radical oxidation lead to the degeneration of cells at a molecular level. If repair or replacement mechanisms are not forthcoming, then cell death is inevitable. The deleterious effect of these reactions can be counteracted upon, if not completely halted, by consuming products containing vitamins A, C, D and E and also β-carotene, chlorophyll and other free radical quenchers. Intense radiation can rupture phosphodiester bonds in one or both strands of DNA. This type of breakage causes a sudden decrease in molecular weight which may or may not be one of the contributing factors that lead to serious malignancy such as cancer.

Chemicals that are ingested can have damaging effect on various parts of the body such as the kidney and the brain. Many organic compounds like anthracene, their derivatives and benzopyrene can be carcinogenic. Most of these aromatic compounds are found in coal tar. Cigarette smoking produces tar which causes papilloma and squamous cell carcinoma. The metabolites formed during interaction with harmful agents, are either removed from the body or catabolized by the host cells. In the case of metals and metallic salts, immunoglobulins form complexes and in the case where the material is inert, it is opsonized or walled off.

Enzymes which control many reactions, can be easily inactivated by several mechanisms. Heavy metallic ions such as arsenic, lead and mercury, can form complex stable salts with -SH groups of the enzymes. Oxidation of enzymes leads to the formation of disulfide linkages thus resulting in the destruction of their functionality. Normal genetic unit of operation is very critical to the cell's homeostasis. Any mutation or chromosomal aberration caused by any agent, may result in the loss of a specific enzyme or even worse in the threat to the very survival of the cell. There are many diseases caused by the deficiency of enzymes and are transmitted by recessive genes.

Pathogenic bacteria and viruses attack mucous membranes that are continually flushed with the products of immune responses. These antibodies are released by the resident cells in response to antigenic stimulation at the mucous surfaces. Viruses are submicroscopic particles which contain genetic material in the form of RNA and DNA (not both) and have protein covering on it. In some cases, the protein covering is surrounded by another coating of carbohydrates and lipids. Viruses replicate their own nucleic acids and contain only those enzymes that are essential to invade the host cell. They are specific in the cell they infect. They fall into two categories: one which causes cell death and the other which triggers the DNA replication thus forming tumor. Some
12

viruses remain dormant in the cells for their entire life, but when the immune system of the host body is depleted, they can cause disease. Viruses are responsible for several types of diseases such as influenza, mumps, measles, disorders of the nervous system and even cancer. Secretory immunoglobulins and enzymes protect the mucosal surfaces by preventing the attachment of bacteria and viruses to the epithelial linings. The initial step in contracting disease involves the colonization of mucosal surfaces.

Most of the diseases are caused either by malnutrition or chronic starvation. Malnutrition usually occurs when the body lacks proper nutrients. Dietary proteins in the food are needed to make proteins in the body during growth period. Proteins not only make structural components of the cells but also enzymes that regulate a vast range of chemical reactions that we call metabolism. Starvation results from lack of nourishment. In acute starvation the body draws energy from its own tissues especially from the adipose tissues. Some of the fat is also degraded to produce essential nutrients for certain tissue that need them. When the remaining reserve of fats are exhausted, the body draws energy from the essential protein-containing tissues. At this stage, the affected body's condition begins to deteriorate. There is a decrease in blood pressure; the body becomes weak and limp and then death soon follows. In chronic starvation multiple deficiencies may appear due to lack of proteins, lipids, vitamins and minerals. There are many diseases associated with chronic starvation.

Terms:

Congenital	*Infectious*	*Inherited*
Allergic	*Autoimmune*	*Molecular*
Metabolic	*Neoplastic*	*Necrosis*

Psychosomatic	Alteration	Infrared
Iatrogenic	Radiation	UV
Dissociation	Chemical bonds	X-rays
Ionizing particles	Chromosomes	Epoxy
Free radical units	Cyclization	Hydroxy
Hydrogen transfer	Chain extension	Aromatic
Cross linking	Benzopyrene	Metabolites
Squamous cell	Catabolized	Bacteria
Immunoglobulins	Carcinoma	Arsenic
Disulfide linkage	Opsonized	Lead
Molecular weight	Homeostatis	Mercury
Peroxy radical units	Carcinogenic	Enzymes
Carboxylic acid	Antibodies	Mumps
Free radical oxidation	β- carotene	Chlorophyll
Phosphodiester bonds	Malnutrition	Measles
Molecular weight	Anthracene	Papilloma
Chronic starvation	Nervous system	Inert
Genetic unit operation	Homeostatis	Viruses
Recessive genes	Host cells	Tumor
Immune response	Nervous system	Influenza
Antigenic stimulation	Resident cells	Secretory

4   Development of Hypothesis

Cells become dysfunctional when their chemical structures or functions are altered or modified.

Mechanism of Aging and Pathogenesis

In this section the fundamentals of aging and pathogenesis will be discussed briefly. Aging itself and age related disorders are degenerative in nature. They may be caused either by depletion of proteins and lipids or by modification in chemical structure of cell proteins and lipids. Depletion or modification or both can be either of enzymes, of immunoglobulins or structural components of a tissue, an organ, an organ system or of the body as a whole. Protein depletion can be due to several reasons: the insufficient secretion of proteins by the cells, disruption or lack of continual supply of raw materials such as amino acids, genetic components, lipids, minerals, vitamins, oxygen and water to the cell. For this reason the cell is either sick or genetically mutated (somatic). For instance, uncontrolled proliferation of immune cells against antigens can deplete the body of proteins as well as specific lipids and therefore makes it more vulnerable to infection. Protein loss can affect protein/lipid ratio in a cell thus affecting its integrity- from cell performance to cell death. Loss of myelin sheath from the axons of neurons may lead to many diseases of the nervous system.

The chemical characteristics of a healthy tissue differs considerably from an unhealthy tissue. The latter either

15

appears depleted, rarefied or swollen. Modified proteins have been found in extracellular matrix and have been implicated in such diseases as swelling of blood vessels, thymus, lymph nodes, glomerular membrane in the kidney, arachnoid membrane, alveolar walls, cornea or in other parts of the body where epithelial surfaces are involved. These modified proteins have sugar moieties that are highly carboxylated or sulfated. They have inherent tendency to swell and form polyanions.

The present hypothesis is that the higher the number of sugar or carbohydrate moieties on the protein core, the higher the oxidation level of that protein structure. In layman's terms, it means that particular protein structure is oxidized or burnt and has an altered functionality. The basic assumption is that once the protein structure is affected, the dysfunction of that particular organ is inevitable. Simply put, individuals affected with cancer, chronic inflammation, obesity, skin ailments and high blood pressure are at higher oxidation level than those individuals with a healthy constitution. Lipids which play a critical role in membrane make up and its function, can be modified like proteins by sugar molecules.

Sugar molecules can interact with proteins in two ways: enzymatically and non-enzymatically. This process of interaction between glucose and protein is known as glycosylation or glycation. Enzymatic glycosylation leads to the formation of proteoglycans. Various types of glycosaminoglycans have been isolated from the extracellular matrix of the connective tissues. Some of the major components are chondroitin sulfate, heparin, heparan sulfate, hyaluronic acid and keratan sulfate. High levels of glycosaminoglycans have also been found in many tumors cells. These proteoglycans may be phenotype alteration in cancer cells. On the other hand non-enzymatic interaction of

16

proteins with glucose can result in the formation of glycosylated proteins. In this typical reaction, the aldehyde group of glucose molecules reacts with the amino group of protein to form Schiff's base product. The concentration of Schiff's base products is a function of the concentration of glucose in the cell. The greater the glycosylation, the higher the oxidation state of the protein under consideration. Glucose interacts with proteins by breaking protein-protein bonds. The modified protein has physical properties entirely different from the native proteins. Such type of interactions can be best understood in terms of cohesive energy density, but because of its highly complex nature there will be no attempt to delve into this subject.

As previously described, radiation of any kind can rupture cell-cell bonds and chemical bonds of DNA, lipids and proteins thereby creating free radical species. These species are highly paramagnetic in nature. They have the tendency to rearrange themselves to form more stable structures. If the chain length is sufficient enough, they can undergo cyclization or intermolecular crosslinking. They can combine with oxygen to form peroxy radicals which can finally lead to the formation of carboxylic acids. Broken down supramolecular structures lead to low molecular weight segments. This is turn causes lesions that result in a positive change in entropy.

Viruses are submicroscopic particles that initiate a unique type of oxidation by replicating their own genetic material to infect a host/body. This type of oxidation is exceedingly rapid and host cells are destroyed in such undefined magnitude. The virus host relation can vary widely ranging from benign co-existence to massive destructive dominance. The ultimate outcome is the destruction of cell-cell bonds or cell-cell cohesiveness which is similar to the effect induced by malnutrition and starvation.

17

All these processes such as dissociation, free radical oxidation, autoxidation, bacterial and viral infection, malnutrition and starvation are degenerative in nature and can cause cascade type of oxidation of cell components such as cell membranes, organelles, regulatory proteins and even genes.

Reduction - Oxidation Cycle

The human body like any other living organism works on reduction-oxidation mechanism. Oxidation reactions are crucial for generating energy within the cell for life processes. The free radical oxidation described in an earlier section differs from enzymatic type of oxidation. The former generates heat in the body whereas enzymatic type of oxidation produces molecules of high energy potential like adenosine triphosphate (ATP). These molecules are produced from the reducing equivalents such as NADH and FADH in the presence of oxygen in a special mitochondrial matrix, by the oxidation of amino acids, fatty acids and glucose in tricarboxylic cycle. Many chemical compounds that are so essential to the life cycle of the cell are made by the process of synthesis that requires high energy molecules and not from heat provided by free radical oxidation.

Though oxidation is the basis of life itself, yet equally important is the continual supply of reductants to preserve the dynamic state of reduction-oxidation cycle without oxidizing the delicate genetic machinery (DNA → m-RNA → Proteins). If all the reductants are exhausted, the reduction-oxidation cycle comes to a halt. Overoxidation can damage tissues, organs and organ systems. The question arises what kind of reducing components should be consumed in the diet that are

18

so essential to the preservation of life. The answer appears to be saturated fats. The highest reduction potential that can be achieved by a living organism is from saturated fats.

Terms

Depletion   *Modification*   *Polyanions*
Myelin sheath   *Heparin*   *NADH, FADH*
Extracellular matrix   *Thymus*   *Alveolar*
Lymph nodes   *Proteoglycan*   *Glycation*
Glomerular   *Cell-cell bond*   *Reductants*
Genetic machinery   *Keratan sulfate*   *Paramagnetic*
Oxidation level   *Heparan sulfate*   *Glycosylation*
Chronic inflammation   *Hyaluronic acid*   *Protocol*
Glycosaminoglycan   *Chondroitin sulfate*   *Schiff's base*
Glycosylated protein   *Cohesive energy density*
Supramolecular structure   *Cell-cell cohesiveness*
Adenosine triphosphate   *Reduction-oxidation cycle*

5 Mystifying Molecules

Cells follow the basic laws of growth.
Any disturbance in their growth mechanism may lead to pathogenesis.

Carbohydrates and fats or lipids are called mystifying molecules because their roles in relation to growth factor has not been explored even though we humans consume these molecules daily. It is the purpose of this chapter to bring into focus some of the mysteries these unique molecules possess.

Carbohydrates and fats are two diverse molecules with entirely diverse functions. By comparing their chemical structures, it becomes evident that saturated fats have more hydrogen atoms than carbohydrates. On the basis of oxygen contents, one molecule of stearic acid $C_{18}H_{36}O_2$ contains two atoms of oxygen whereas glucose $C_6H_{12}O_6$ carries six atoms of oxygen. On carbon content basis, the ratio of oxygen between them is 1:9. From this simple analysis it can be inferred that glucose is more oxidized than stearic acid. Glucose is a highly reactive molecule because it contains one aldehyde group that can easily condense with lipids and proteins to form glycolipids, glycosylated proteins and proteoglycans. These resulting molecules have unique characteristic to attract water in contrast to stearic acid which has the inherent tendency to repel water.

Because of its unique reactivity with lipids and proteins, glucose is hereby defined as an oxidant as compared to lipids and proteins which are termed as reductants. The question is being raised, what is an oxidant? An oxidant is a compound that tends to oxidize cell components such as lipids, nucleic acids and proteins. It is also known as electron acceptor.

20

In order for oxidation to take place, a corresponding compound should be present to release electrons. Such compounds are known as reductants; it means that they have the tendency to reduce cell components. Thus in living organisms, oxidation process involves the removal of hydrogen atoms as compared to reduction process which often involves the addition of hydrogen atoms.

As mentioned previously, lipids form membranes which enclose cell, cell organelles and genetic material. These membranes not only provide the housing for cell components but they also create strong electrochemical potential barriers. This electron transport system is unique in that the electrons are released and passed on to the next molecules. In a dynamic system like human cell, there is a constant turn over of electrons and protons especially when the new cells are being generated at an enormous rate. Since man is not solar powered like plants, he has to rely heavily on materials formed by solar radiation.

Thus cells with saturated fatty acids form formidable barrier against oxidative degradation and prolong the life span of the cell. In contrast the membranes of unsaturated fatty acids provide poor protection to the cells and their components. They have the tendency to undergo oxidation and form intermediates that can react with DNA, regulatory proteins and structural components. This causes lesions in the cells through which oxygen can diffuse easily. This is another route through which amino acids, enzymes, antibodies and genetic materials are oxidized. In such cases autoxidation should be taken into consideration. Thus natural saturated fatty acids are termed as healthy fats because they provide constant supply of electrons that enables the cellular machinery to run efficiently.

Lipids constitute about 40 percent of the organic matter in the body. Membranes control the flow of information between the cells and their immediate environment. Protein chains are embedded in a lipid bilayer. These chains act as pumps, gates, receptors and energy transducers. It is these protein molecules with carbohydrate moieties that confer individuality to each of the cell. Some of the other functions of lipids in the body are to;

* act as composite for the durability of the cell;
* act as lubricant for epithelial layers of the skin and mucosa;
* act as effective emulsifiers for digestive materials;
* act as insulator and also as energy source for the body;
* act as antibacterial and antifungal agents for the skin;
* provide protection to many organs in the body; and enhance the phagocytic potential of immune surveillance network

On a gram to gram basis fat provides twice as much the amount of energy as glucose. Fats enter into chemical reactions which are less harmful to cell components than carbohydrates. Fats also carry vitamins such as A, D, E and K.

Terms:

Stearic acid   *Electron*
Electrochemical potential   *Vitamin A*
Electron transport system   *Autoxidation*
Unsaturated fatty acid   *Intermediate*
Regulatory proteins   *Emulsifier*
Immune surveillance   *Antibacterial*
Phagocytic potential   *Vitamin D*
Antifungal   *Vitamin K*

6   Regulated Cell Growth

Healing mechanisms become slow or affected when cells are deprived of essential constituents.

(Kakar)

In most chronic illnesses, either there is a rapid loss in cell density of a particular tissue or organ or modification in cell structure or its functions. Since cells follow the basic laws of growth, any disturbance in their growth cycle may lead to atrophy, hyperplasia, dysplasia, neoplasia or any other undefined disorder. The logical approach to cure age related or degenerative illnesses, is to create a proper environment for cell growth. Even a sick cell can be revived by nourishing with appropriate nutrients such as amino acids, nucleic acid components, fats, mineral and vitamins and can be brought to a dynamic state of reproduction. Cell revival will lead to more cells which lead to the formation of sufficient amount of proteins needed for various functions in the body. Some of these proteins may be used for structural components by associating with lipids, but majority of them will be used as enzymes that are needed as catalysts to carry out different chemical reactions in the body.

For proper cell growth, collagen support is essential and contact between the cells is needed for differentiation and maturation. Collagen formed by the cells should be of specific chemical constitution to achieve proper cell adhesion between the cells as well as between the collagen and the cells. Collagen studded with large number of sugar molecules exhibit poor adhesive characteristics as compared to collagen that has fewer sugar moieties. Presence of these modified structures in the body denotes deficiency in the levels of various enzymes such as hydrolases and reductases.

©

Experimental Model:

In this section I will discuss in detail how food constituents such as carbohydrates, fats, nucleic acid components and proteins that we consume on a daily basis, can react with one another in the body to give rise to biofunctional and non-biofunctional structures in the body. Biofunctional structures are essential for generating cells, tissues, organs and organ systems, whereas non-biofunctional components such as inert, crosslinked, reactive species are harmful and indicate the absence of enzymatic activity. The following study was conducted to investigate the effect of food constituents alone and in combination at various concentrations on the human body. The object of this study was to find a region where optimum yield of biofunctional molecules takes place.

Human body for its survival needs several components such as dietary proteins, dietary nucleic acid components, fats carbohydrates, minerals, vitamins, oxygen and water. The manner in which we consume food constituents can have considerable effect on the status of our health. The response Y which is defined as the status of health, can be written as a function (f) of

$$Y = f (P)(N)(F)(C)(M)(V)(O)(W)$$

at constant temperature   (1)

24

where (P), (N), (F), (C), (M), (V), (O) and (W) are the respective concentrations of dietary proteins, nucleic acids components, fats, carbohydrates, minerals, vitamins, oxygen and water.

Certain assumptions have to be made before this design can be used effectively. The first assumption is that the concentrations of oxygen and water remain constant despite their interaction with many components in the body. The second assumption is that vitamins and minerals are integral part of natural food constituents and third assumption is that proteins and nucleic acid components are inseparable and will be regarded as one unit. The equation (1) is reduced to

$$Y \ = \ f(P.N)(F)(C) \tag{2}$$

The response Y becomes a function of protein/nucleic acid components, fats and carbohydrates. Figure 6-1 shows the interaction between these food constituents at various concentrations:

constituent X_1 = carbohydrates

constituent X_2 = natural saturated fats

constituent X_3 = dietary protein/nucleic acid components

From this figure it is evident that the respective concentrations of X_1, X_2 and X_3 are zero at respective points K, L and M. Line $X_1 X_3$ represents the interaction between carbohydrates

25

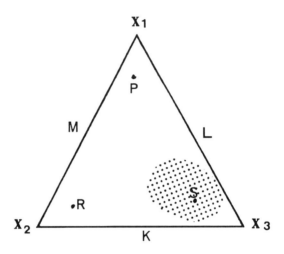

Figure 6-1:   Three Component Mixture Model

and proteins/nucleic acid components which gives rise to the formation of glycosylated proteins such as proteoglycans, glycoproteins and glycosylated nucleic acid components at various concentrations. The line X_1X_2 shows the interaction between carbohydrates and fats or lipids which results in the formation of lipoglycans and glycolipids. The interaction between lipids and proteins leads to the formation of proteolipids and lipoproteins and is represented by the line X_2X_3. Any point in between the triangle represents the interaction between three constituents such as carbohydrates, lipids and proteins at various concentrations. The situation becomes even more complicated when the action of dissociation and oxygen comes into interplay.

Thus the food constituents we consume interact with one another in the body to form glycosylated lipoproteins, lipoproteoglycans, glycosylated proteolipids, glycosylated proteins, glycosylated nucleic acid components and glycosylated lipids depending upon the way we consume food. Some of the components such as glycosylated proteins and glycosylated and crosslinked fats are non-biofunctional and their presence in excessive amount in the body denotes malignancies. But other components such as natural saturated fats, proteins and lipoproteins of high molecular weight or high density lipoproteins which are biofunctional, are essential for cell formation and cell-cell interaction. When a lipoprotein of high molecular weight is highly glycosylated or in other words oxidized, its density drops considerably. The other components that also accumulate in the body are the intermediate products of autoxidation of proteins, lipids and carbohydrates.

Let us examine this model more closely. For example, the point S in Figure 6-1 represents the situation, where X_1 = 10% , X_2 = 10% and X_3 = 80%. A healthy response can be obtained when the ratio of carbohydrates, natural saturated fats and dietary proteins/nucleic acid components is kept 1:1:8.

Point P represents a very unhealthy response where the ratio of the constituents is 8: 1: 1. Individuals consuming food constituents in this ratio over a long period, may acquire diseases of extracellular matrix. These individuals have eroded epithelial layers (skin and mucosal linings) and have carbohydrates moieties exposed which become attractive sites for antigens containing similar structures such as bacteria and cancerous tissues. The effect can be more pronounced when polyunsaturated fats are substituted instead of saturated fats. Ailments such as allergies, bronchitis, common cold, chronic infection, chronic inflammation, hay fever, heart attack, ulcer and high blood pressure are related to eroded epithelial layers. Prolonged symptoms may lead to arthritis, osteoporosis and rheumatoid arthritis. Diseases related to aging, bone marrow and autoimmune syndromes pertain to this region.

Point R represents a situation which is rather impractical. Diet rich in natural saturated fats (beyond 30%) is indigestible. In my studies natural saturated fats have been found to be extremely useful in reversing aging and many degenerative disorders. There are many diseases related to accumulation of lipids in the body. These lipid deposits are either oxidized, partially glycosylated or crosslinked structures that the body is unable to utilize due to lack of enzymes. Accumulated glycolipids become attractive sites for colonization of gram negative bacteria.

The shaded area in the figure where the amount of carbohydrates is low and that of proteins is high with regulated amount of natural saturated fats, appears to be suitable for curing many types of chronic and degenerative ailments. Though this manuscript is confined to aging and age
28

related illnesses, it seems appropriate to mention at this stage some of my findings about common illnesses. During the course of my investigation, I found that the body becomes resistant to infection. Repeated episodes of common cold were reduced to much fewer ones resulting in slight headaches and restlessness without fever. Chronic sinusitis and chronic bronchitis disappeared in the course of a few months. It appears that this much time is needed to deglycosylate the body to a desired level of glycosylation against future infection. It is generally assumed that a person is cured of infection, if the episode of infection is over. In reality it is hardly the case. For a body to be cured of infection the underlying cause has to be eliminated.

All ingredients used in this study were fresh with the exception of refined carbohydrates and vegetable oils. The source of carbohydrates was unbleached flour, rice and refined sugar. The source of proteins/nucleic acid components was eggs, fish, red meat and vegetables. These ingredients were also the source of minerals and vitamins. The source of saturated fats was animal fats, butter and coconut milk. These were also the source of oil soluble vitamins and free radical quenchers. Additional source of water soluble vitamins and minerals was fresh fruits. No supplementary or synthetic vitamins or minerals were included in this study.

The shaded area is designated as cell growth region where regulated cell growth takes place. In order to examine the validity of the result, monounsaturated fats were substituted for natural saturated fats. Surprisingly, the symptoms which were last resolved in a previous study appeared early during this trial and the results were more pronounced with polyunsaturated fats. It has become evident that a healthy body becomes extremely sensitive to harmful and unfamiliar substances. It is deduced from this study that a healthy body tends to keep its integrity as against a diseased body that has a tendency to destroy itself. It is quite clear that the types of fats consumed have a crucial role to play in keeping the integrity of the cell. Cell membranes composed of monounsaturated and polyunsaturated lipids tend to disintegrate faster than membranes of saturated lipids against oxidative and biological stresses. These cells have less chance to survive, proliferate, differentiate and mature than the cells of natural saturated fats. Maturation is an essential phase in cell life cycle because at this stage, cells are able to produce specific proteins for various functions in the body. Early disappearance of large number of cells leads to the accumulation of disintegrated fragments of cells, which if not removed can cause clogging of blood vessels and other complications. Due to rapid loss of cells some organs develop lesions which never heal and if this situation is continued for a long period of time it may lead to the loss of an organ.

One can safely assume that a close relationship exists between the degree of saturation of lipids and the shape of the cell membranes. A closed examination of a cell structure reveals that the hereditary material is protected in a double walled membrane. This degree of protection is essential because of the sensitive nature of DNA, enzymes and regulatory proteins to oxidation. Only saturated fats can provide maximum potential barrier to cell organelles and nuclear material against oxidation and thus contribute to the life of the cell.

Polyunsaturated fats at any level can cause serious immunologic disorders such as threatening respiratory infection and various types of cancers. Excessive consumption over a long period of time leads to arthritis, back pain, osteoporosis, pathologic fractures, stiff knees, and other severe types of bone related disorders. Early symptoms include cartilage erosion leading to bone spur formation.

30

These deformities may lead to immobilization. Most of these deformities are related to autoimmune syndrome. The ability of NK cells and macrophages to kill bacteria becomes sluggish and the activity of many immune cells decline substantially because of insufficient lysosomal activity in these cells.

Terms:

Regulated cell growth   *Growth cycle*   *Cell density*
Atrophy   *Hyperplasia*   *Metaplasia*
Dysplasia   *Neoplasia*   *Collagen*
Adhesion   *Hydrolases*   *Reductases*
Optimum yield   *Function*   *Interaction*
Biofunctional   *Bronchitis*   *Sinusitis*
Osteoporosis   *Differentiate*   *Maturation*
Proliferate   *Deglycosylate*   *NK Cells*
Non-biofunctional   *Glycosylated lipoprotein*
Lipoproteoglycan   *Glycosylated proteolipid*
Glycosylated nucleic acid   *High density lipoprotein*
Cell-cell interaction   *Gram negative bacteria*
Autoimmune system   *Rheumatoid arthritis*
Monounsaturated fats   *Polyunsaturated fats*
Immunologic disorders   *Macrophages*
Lysosomal activity

7 Mathematical Model for Healing

Cells have the unique ability to cure illnesses provided they are nourished properly.
  (Kakar)

Through series of studies the following empirical relationship was developed which summarizes all the facts discussed so far. This equation explains the relationship between the growth factor and necrosis factors and their relationship with genetic machinery for forming a new generation of genes.

©

$$\text{OK RecoveryFactor} = \frac{(SF)\,(P.N)}{(C)}\; G_k \,/\, m$$

at constant temperature (3)

where G_k is called Kakar genetic constant and represents the inherited genetic machinery, m is the variable and indicates the extent of mutation induced in the genetic material. Terms (SF), (P.N) and (C) denote respective concentrations of dietary natural saturated fats, protein/nucleic acid components and dietary carbohydrates. Segment (SF) (P.N) of equation (3) is related to growth factor and through genetic machinery strictly regulates the cell growth, cell-cell differentiation and cell-cell interaction or cohesiveness. Term (C) is related to necrosis factors. Excessive consumption of carbohydrates such as glucose or starch makes cells sensitive to external as well as internal stimuli by breaking the cell-cell bonds. Other risk factors that can damage the cell-cell cohesiveness, are bacteria, chemical agents, temperature, pressure, radiation, physical and emotional stress. It is evident from this equation that recovery factor or immune level has direct correlation with growth factor and inverse correlation with necrosis factor. Further analysis of this equation reveals that factor (SF)/(C) is related to reduction/oxidation potential. For efficient protein synthesis by the cells, there ought to exist potential barrier between the nucleus and the nuclear membrane, DNA and RNA, synthesized proteins and the vesicle, cell organelles and the cytoplasmic membrane. In many chronic or degenerative disorders an unusual situation arises when the body utilizes factor (P.N)/(C) for reduction-oxidation cycle due to lack of natural saturated fats. In such cases body derives its energy from protein/nucleic acid and glucose interaction to meet its immediate demand. This type of situation is related to autoimmune syndrome and should be avoided because of unpleasant results. In equation (3) the terms (SF) and (P.N) may be added together for practical application under special circumstances. The above equation assumes the following form.

©

$$\text{OK Recovery Factor} \; = \; \frac{(SF) + (P.N)}{(C)} \; G_k \, /m$$

or   (4)

Immune Level

This model can be used as a useful guide for curing many chronic disorders and for understanding pathogenesis and healing. For accurate study the effect of other necrosis factors must be taken into account.

Effect of carbohydrates on membrane receptors

Cells like humans communicate and interact with one another through surface receptors or antennas. If they cooperate and communicate effectively, they can form dense and coherent organs that are impregnable by any virus or bacteria. The effective communication is largely dependent upon the chemical composition of surface receptors of the cells. Cells like humans also acquire specialization in their field. Cell-cell interaction is of fundamental importance in cell differentiation. Cell differentiation is a process by which identical cells adopt specialized functions such as muscle cells that contract. It has been noticed in my recent studies that receptors with few sugar moieties have better adhesion to the cells with similar type receptors. They form organs with high degree of cohesiveness. The tendency of carbohydrates is to break the cell-cell cohesiveness and cell-cell interaction. This results in the formation of loosely held swollen mass of identical undifferentiated cells. Organs containing such structures are highly inflamed and susceptible to infection and other harmful agents. In most cases they give the appearance of tumor or independent growth (Figure 7-1).

Effect of carbohydrates on DNA segments

In equation (3) m is the variable that indicates the extent of mutation induced in the genetic machinery. Since carbohydrates are internal oxidants, their consumption in excessive amount

34

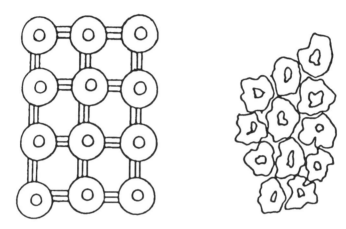

Figure 7-1: Normal cell-cell cohesiveness is shown
on the left and the loss of cohesiveness
on the right. It shows the development
of neoplasm with irregular shape.

can affect DNA segments of the genes in various ways. Glucose can cause excessive production of ATP molecules rather than deoxy ATP molecules that are needed for the formation of new genes. When deoxyribose molecules are not available, the new strands of genes will have ribose as the sugar unit instead of deoxy ribose. These segments are deleted or in other words oxidized and become attractive sites for virus for further oxidation. Glucose can react enzymatically and nonenzymatically with regulatory proteins thus affecting the delicate process of regulated cell growth. Further dissociation and oxidation of DNA segments can lead to the formation of complex cyclic or crosslinked structures that are non-biofunctional thereby denoting malignancies in the cell. Thus carbohydrates can be villain if not properly managed.

Immune level is defined as the ratio between the growth factor and necrosis factor. Therefore various immune levels can be attained by changing the concentration of carbohydrates and other necrosis factors with respect to the types of dietary fats, proteins and nucleic acid components.

Human population is classified into three categories based on immune levels.

Immunodeficient: when growth factor is less than necrosis factors. growth factor < necrosis factors

Immunocompromising: when growth factor is equal or slightly greater than necrosis factors. growth factor = necrosis factors

36

| Immunocompetent | when growth factor is greater than necrosis factors. |
| | growth factor > necrosis factors |

It becomes evident that aging and disease formation processes are related to the dynamic of growth and inflammatory processes. Growth factor which involves protein synthesis, is mediated through release of variety of hormones such as growth hormones, sex hormones, regulatory hormones, etc. These hormones are of two types: steroid and peptide. Steroid hormones such as aldosterone, cortisols, estradiol, progesterone and testosterone are derived from cholesterol and saturated fatty acids, whereas growth hormones, prolactin, epinephrine, norepinephrine, dopamine, melanine and thyroxin are derived from amino acids or dietary proteins. Central nervous system which houses hypothalamus and pituitary glands, strictly controls the release of these hormones, which is induced by many factors. These precursors trigger genes in many cell types (Figure 8-1) to produce tissues, organs and organ systems through various mechanisms. Thus healthy gene expression involves a series of complex reactions, which requires integrated interaction of all cell types.

Terms:

Aldosterone	*Dopamine*	*Immune level*
ATP	*Epinephrine*	*Mutation*
Cholesterol	*Estradiol*	*Prolactin*
Cortisol	*Growth hormones*	*Pituitary gland*
Deleted segments	*Hypothalamus*	*Progesterone*
Deoxy ATP	*Immunocompetent*	*Steroid*
Deoxyribose	*Immunodeficient*	*Testosterone*
Immunocompromising		*Undifferentiated cells*

8 Dynamics of Growth Factor

Natural saturated fats are the strongest reductants that biological world can produce.

(Kakar)

What is so unique about living things that make them emerge, grow, survive and die? The answer to these complex questions may be simpler than you have in mind. If we analyze the structural components of living cells, it immediately becomes clear that all have relatively higher reduction potential than the environment in which they live. The only structural material that can create such a strong electrochemical potential barrier is the delicate membrane. Since the genetic engine is a perpetual machinery which plays a crucial role in the control and direction of cellular growth and reproduction, the membrane becomes a highly labile system for the transfer of electrons. Thus constant supply of lipids becomes essential especially, when the new cells are being generated.

Aging of Genes

It is an accepted fact that the linear order of nucleotides in DNA segment determines the sequencing of amino acids in a protein. This therefore is the determinant for protein's structure and its function. Any slight modification in its linearity and its chemical structure can result in catastrophic

38

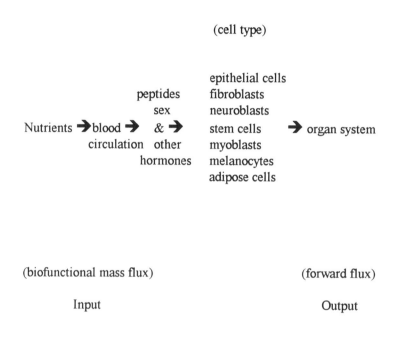

(cell type)

Figure 8-1: General diagram shows the conversion of biofunctional mass into forward flux of growth factor to sustain an organ. It also shows how hormones released by central nervous system, stimulate the growth of various types of cells.

outcome. Thus genes like any macromolecule, are liable to dissociation, glycosylation, oxidation, and other degenerative processes. The concept of growth factor actually originated from my earlier work with silk worms, their cells and their sequence of nucleotides and later with humans. By this unique technique mutated genes could be repaired, revived/reduced and brought back to healthy reproductive state by replicating them in vivo or in a reduced environment. Forward flux of growth factor that I have stated below, is the most powerful mechanism that is operative in all mammalian cells on this planet.

©

Kakar Forward Flux of Growth Factor in Rejuvenation and Healing Mechanism

Human cells are continuously utilizing raw materials in form of nutrients such as amino acids derived from various specific tissues of animals or plants, natural fats, minerals, vitamins and water to make new sets of genes and cell components.

$$\text{Ideal Growth Factor} = (SF)(P.N) \rightarrow \circlearrowleft G_k \qquad (5)$$
(gene expression)

Where genetic machinery G_k is made up of several sets of genes. Each gene which contains sequence of nucleotides, codes for a specific polypeptide or protein. Transcription in genes is controlled by release of various neuroproteins. For healthy neuromusculovascular network constant release of enzymes, globular proteins, hormones and amino acids becomes essential.

40

Equation (5) explains a unique relationship between biofunctional mass and the ideal growth factor. The scheme of administering nutrients into the cell is shown in Figure 8-1. Each cell acts as an extruder as well as a reactor. It is the integrated interaction of all the cell types that sustains an organ system. As the nutrients flow into the cells, a concentration graident or concentration flux (in terms of enzymes, growth hormones that control the production of structural and functional proteins, immunoglobulins, etc.) develops which is facilitated by blood circulation. Deficiency and change in the composition of any ingredient can cause change in growth flux. This forward flux is very crucial to body's survival mechanism and significantly contributes to healing mechanism. It differs from regular healing mechanism where the damaged tissues are replaced by identical but new tissues.

Thus layers after layers of forward flux are constantly generated to replace the old ones. This virtually happens in every organ system of the body but the rate of generation may differ from one organ system to another. This is the way body tends to rejuvenate itself and tries to get rid of bacteria, toxins and viruses provided the flux is of proper chemical constitution and composition. The rate and quality of forward flux is largely dependent upon the food constituents that are fed to the body and the types of lipids deposited in the bone marrow and bony tissues. Diseases usually develop when the forward flux is either highly glycosylated, oxidized or virtually non-existent. The later situation usually develops when the body is either starved or subjected to malnutrition. Instead of generating a new flux, body uses its own resources to keep itself alive. Lesions develop in many organs of the body due to breakdown and depletion of cells. In extreme cases organs regress. They become rarefied, stiff, brittle and lose their functionality. A forward flux of high reducion potential may

41

be generated by using methodology described in page 60 which heals lesions and chronic infection. It repairs/replaces glycosylated/oxidized genes and oxidized structures of many organs and brings the body from immunodeficient level to immunocompetent level.

The general facts about growth factor are summarized below;

*   nutrition and genes go hand in hand. Genetic
        machinery is dysfunctional without nutrition
        and without genes there is no life;

*   growth factor involves the interaction of reducing
        components such as natural fats containing
        saturataed/unsaturated lipids, amino acids or dietary
        proteins/nucleic acid components with genetic
        machinery. It repairs/replaces mutated genes
        and generates new ones as situation demands.

*   growth factor is a reduction as well as growth
        process whereas necrosis factors involve
        depletion or/and oxidation process/es;

*   growth factor has unique antibacterial, antifungal,
        antiinflammatory, antiparasitic and antiviral
        characteristics;

*   growth factor helps cell-cell interaction and
        cell-cell cohesiveness, whereas necrosis
        factors undermine this cohesiveness;

*   diseases develop when growth factor is inhibited
        or interfered by any mechanism in the body;

*   all illnesses acute, infectious, or chronic denote

progressive oxidation of various parts of the body
and through growth factor they may be healed and

*   growth factor of various oxidation potentials may be
generated by consuming refined carbohydrates,
minerals and processed lipids other than natural fats
which may or may not contribute to adequate healing
and lead to abnormal and poor cell growth.

Growth factor may cure many disorders related to
cardiovascular, central nervous system, immune system and
musculoskeletal network.

Cardiovascular Disorders

Cardiovascular disorders include a wide range of diseases that
affect heart, and blood vessels. Common symptoms include
chest pains, palpitation and shortness of breath. Several risk
factors such as diabetes, hypertension, high serum cholesterol
levels, infection, lipid dysfunction and smoking have been
identified. These factors may also be responsible for clogging,
hardening and narrowing of arteries due to deposition of fatty
materials containing cholesterol, calcium and other minerals.
In emergency cases, where the coronary arteries are blocked
and heart does not receive sufficient blood supply, coronary
bypass may be warranted.

Individuals of all ages are prone to heart attacks due to
varying reasons. Some of the cardiovascular ailments may be
related to high levels of calcium and iron in serum caused by
malfunction in muscleoskeletal network or it may also be
simply due to high amount of dietary intake of calcium and

iron which results in the displacement of potassium. Cardiovascular disorders among most of the elderly may be due to erosion of blood vessel linings, bones, bone marrow, connective tissues and neuromuscular junctions. The fundamental reason behind this may be the loss of microscopic and macroscopic collagens that hold virtually every tissue and organ in the body. Presence of high level of low density lipoproteins and cholesterol in serum may indicate that the food being consumed contains high levels of oxidants and does not contribute to healthy growth factor. Chronic high blood pressure is a classical example where growth factor is exceeded by necrosis factors. Cells are dying at a more rapid rate than they are produced. There are not enough healthy cells available to conduct the phagocytic activities. Thus every individual case needs proper analysis and judgment before any proper course of action is executed.

Central Nervous System

Central nervous system includes brain, ears, eyes, spinal cord and peripheral nerves. Input to the nervous system is furnished by the sensory receptors. Brain is the most sensitive organ of the human body and is easily influenced by ideas, emotions, events, chemical agents, pain, drugs, bacteria and viruses and is liable to many disorders. Confused brain syndrome is the most common disorders found not only among the elderly but also among the population of all ages. Disorders such as dizziness, headaches, depression, impaired balance, poor memory, neurosis, phobias, senility, Alzheimer's disease, multiple sclerosis and Parkinson's disease may indicate progressive degeneration of central nervous system.

44

Like any organ system, central nervous system is subject to general process of depletion, dissociation, glycosylation and oxidation. Neurons have high metabolic rates and are extremely sensitive to glucose and oxygen concentration. Degeneration of lipid layers in neurons leads to the accumulation of fibrillar material. These fibrous plaques consist of mainly matted, twisted and interwoven unmyelinted axons. In many cases, myelin sheath that protects nerve fibers of central nervous system, is destroyed and sclerosed patches are formed. Neurons like any other tissues can be grown by using Growth Factor technique and many neural ailments such as, anxiety, Alzheimer's disease, behavioral disorders, depression, paralysis, learning disorders, mood swing, multiple sclerosis, phobias, retinopathy, and several other psychosomatic and visual disorders may be healed.

Musculoskeletal System

Musculoskeletal system is comprised of bones, muscles and joints. Skeleton is a vital supportive structure to an organism. In addition to its support, skeleton has several other functions. It protects soft tissues against external hazards by acting as a shield. It provides anchors for the muscles. These muscles in association with other bone joints, produce locomotion by contraction. Bone is composed of mainly two components, inorganic and organic matrix. Inorganic matrix is mainly of crystals of hydroxy apatite or calcium phosphate whereas the organic matrix is composed chiefly of collagen. Collagen not only forms bones but other supportive structures such as ligaments, tendons, underlying fibril network for skin, blood vessels and teeth and perform many other structural functions in the body. Virtually every organ in the body is penetrated by microscopic and macroscopic collagen. Collagen is related to a family of fibrous proteins which form insoluble fibers of exceptionally high strength. So far twelve types of collagens have been identified. Collagen holds cells and has a major role in the development of all tissues and organs. In order to maintain the physiological functions of tissues and cells, proper regulation of collagen mechanism is of utmost importance. With advancing age, musculoskeletal system undergoes progressive deterioration due to chemical modification of collagen. Many chronic disorders such as arthritis, osteoarthritis, osteoporosis, rheumatoid arthritis, gout, neoplasm of joints, muscular dystrophy and polymyositis develop. Decrease in synthesis of collagen may be another reason for decalcification of bone cells. Healthy bones usually have healthy bone marrow.

The contraction of muscles usually results from sliding motion of two kind of filaments, actin and myosin. Energy for the contraction cycle is derived from the hydrolysis of ATP by calcium dependent ATP enzymes. Relaxation of muscle action is achieved by magnesium ions. Thus contraction and relaxation cycles are controlled by calcium/ magnesium channels. Many muscular disorders are caused by several reasons such as interference with the conduction of motor end plate, loss of motor unit, glycogen storage, loss of enzymes and their activity. Transmission of signals to muscles via neurons is achieved by neuromuscular junctions. Myasthenia gravis is denoted by weakness in voluntary muscles. The weakness arises either due to impaired neuromuscular transmission or due to lack of acetylcholine receptors. It is suggested that the defect could be in the motor end plate. Individuals with myasthenia have hyperthyroidism. Though muscle diseases are very rare, there are more neuromuscular diseases because neurons are involved in every muscular activity. They may be effectively cured by Growth Factor technique.

46

Immune System

The importance of immune system is not realized until the individual falls victim to cancer or faced with life threatening disorders. The field of immunology is quite complex and research activities are underway from many disciplines. Immune system is a kind of defense network that body uses to challenge variety of pathogens and toxins that are present in the environment. Body uses various strategies to resist these agents or antigens that tend to destroy tissues and organs. The ability to resist or combat these agents is termed immunity. Immunity can be adaptive or non-adaptive. The non-adaptive immunity makes the body resistant to certain diseases such as dysentery and viral diseases of animals. In adaptive immune response, body generates antibodies against a particular antigen such as virus. These antibodies can prevent the virus from spreading or entering into the cell. White blood cells are the dynamic units of body's defense mechanism. These cells are of two kinds; with granules and without granules. Cells with granules include neutrophils, eosinophils and basophils. Cells without granules are monocytes, lymphocytes and plasma cells. All these cells use various mechanisms to kill the intruder. Antibodies are also referred to as immunoglobulins. There are at least five different types of immunoglobulins in serum designated as IgG, IgM, IgA, IgD, and IgE. In the serum, IgG is the largest in proportion. This immunoglobulin is directed against infectious agents such as bacteria, viruses and toxins. IgG is responsible for the protection of fetus during maturation of its immune system. IgM is the largest molecule and has ten antibody reaction sites and is important for primary immune response. IgA immunoglobulin is found in secretion such as tears, saliva and mucus of respiratory and digestive tracts. IgE is related to acute allergic responses such

47

as asthma, hay fever and anaphylaxis and helps to protect against parasites. The exact function of IgD immunoglobulin is not known.

The acquired or adaptive immunity is achieved by lymphocytes namely B-cells and T-cells. The B-cells develop in bone marrow (stem cell) and may differentiate into plasma cells which produce antibodies. The T-cells differentiate in thymus and help B-cells to make antibodies. B lymphocytes are related to the humoral response, which neutralizes bacteria and other invaders, whereas T-lymphocytes are related to cell mediated response. In humoral response, the antibodies are secreted by the plasma cells located on the lymph nodes and lymphoid organs and away from the invasion sites, whereas in cell mediated response, the sensitized T-cells travel to the invasion sites and interact with specific antigen. The chemicals released after the interaction of the sensitized T-lymphocytes with specific antigen, can kill cells directly. Some of the chemicals released are chemotactic factors which attract monocytes and neutrophils to the site of attack. Monocytes are converted to giant cells known as macrophages which carry out phagocytic activities. In addition to cytotoxic T-cells, there are other two classes of T-cells known as helper T-cells and suppressor T-cells. These two types of T-cells help to facilitate or suppress the expression of B-cells to produce antibodies. The suppressor T-cells inhibit inappropriate antibody production. The failure of suppresser T-cells to regulate the uncontrolled production of antibodies, leads to an allergic response such as hypersensitivity. In many chronic infectious diseases, even the macrophages that carry out phagocytic activities become infected.

Allergies, anaphylaxis type-I (hay fever), anaphylaxis type II, anaphylaxis type III, anaphylaxis type IV (delayed hyper sensitivity), autoimmune syndrome and AIDS are related to defective immune system and indicate poor regulated cell growth. Equation (3) explains clearly how to accelerate the effective immune response by increasing growth factor and inhibiting the necrosis factors.

Cancer

Cancer is described as dysfunction in cell growth mechanism. It develops when a cell or group of cells do not follow the rules of regulatory cell growth mechanism. Instead, they develop their own existence. A normal cell is committed to cell functions whereas cancer cell is preoccupied with undifferentiated cell growth which leads to tumor formation. Tumor can be either benign or malignant. A benign tumor is slow growing and does not cause secondary growth in a distant location or metastasize. In contrast, malignant tumor is composed of fast growing cells that destroys neighboring tissues and tends to metastasize. Probably there are as many types of cancers as there are organs in the body such as breast, buccal cavity, colon, liver, ovary, pancreas, prostate, throat, uterus etc.

Currently several approaches are being applied to understand the basis of carcinogenesis. Studies such as clinical analysis of tumor cells show that these tumors contain high levels of proteoglycans. The real significance of these materials in extracellular matrix has not been fully explored.

One or many necrosis factors may be involved in cancer formation process which affect the regulated growth process. Equation (3) clearly explains how necrosis factors can

49

mutate genes, affect the cell-cell adhesion or cell-cell interaction. Development of any growth whether benign or malignant on mucosal and epithelial surfaces denotes sharp decline in the levels of healthy adipose tissues and are indicative of slow or sudden oxidative outbursts in an organ or organ system involved. Usually depletion of healthy fatty tissues occurs in areas such as brain, bony tissues, bone marrow cavities, breast, colon, face, lips, lymph nodes, beneath the skin and prostate. These tissues become replaced by non-biofunctional materials. The current tendency is to remove these materials either surgically, by radiotherapy or chemotherapy. The results with chemotherapy have not been very pleasant in many cases because this methodology drastically destroys the very immune system that protects the body against diseases. The logical approach is to create an environment for regulated cell growth. It is envisioned that Growth Factor may take the place of chemotherapy as a possible cure for any illness.

Morbid Obesity

Morbid obesity is another example where growth factor is exceeded by necrosis factors. In this case, the hypothalamus which regulates the feeding mechanism is damaged. Individuals with this condition have large amount of non-biofunctional mass that has the property of attracting large amount of fluid. Their organs are highly glycosylated or burnt and may be healed through Growth Factor technique. These individuals have to generate fibrillar collagen to form bones, bone marrow and muscles rather than extracellular matrix.

Terms:

Genetic engine

Depurination

Nucleotides

Hyperuricemia

Forward Flux

Cardiovascular

Hypertension

Peripheral nerves

Motor end- plate

Hyperthyroidism

Immunoglobulins

Plasma

Antigen

Humoral

Phagocytic

Hypersensitivity

Nucleotides

Catabolism

Azotemia

Uric acid

Extruder

Palpitaion

Cholesterol

Polymyositis

Monocytes

Lymphocytes

Eosinophil

B-cell

Thymus

Macrophages

Anaphylaxis

Metastasize

Chromosomes

Purine

Uremia

Kidney stone

Reactor

Gout

Gradient

Acetylcholine

Granules

Neutrophil

Basophil

T-cells

Antibodies

Cytotoxic

Benign

Malignant

9   Total Healing and Restoration

The genetic machinery that we inherit in the form of a fertilized egg is perpetual .
   (Kakar)

Total healing may be defined as a process of restoring the aged or unhealthy body to its original healthy state. This is exactly opposite to pathogenesis. At this stage it is important to make a distinction between medical treatment and healing. In the case of medical treatment, the process either attacks the symptoms of the illness or assists the healing powers of Nature. This could be easily worked out if the illness is of transient nature, but not so when it comes to chronic or age related illnesses. In the case of healing, the process involves the use of natural food constituents to promote the growth factor.

Factors that cause aging and degenerative disorders are:

*   polluted environment;
*   inactivity;
*   stress including emotional stress;
*   malnutrition;
*   starvation;
*   heavy smoking and drinking;
*   frequent ingestion of prescription and off the counter drugs, minerals and vitamins supplements;
*   excessive sex indulgence under the influence of drugs;

*   excessive masturbation and indiscriminate sex;
*   excessive consumption of refined carbohydrates and
        processed oils and fats;
*   repeated bacterial and viral attacks and
*   interaction with harmful chemicals and parasites.

They either induce alteration in cell structure, cell metabolism, genetic code or in extreme cases cause cell depletion. The induced alterations cause drastic decline in total reduction potential of an organ, organ system or the body as a whole. Most of the degenerative disorders have their origin in the malfunction of autonomic nervous system. Therefore they take longer time to heal ranging from several months to several years. The extent of duration depends upon the degree of damage inflicted on the body and its ability for rejuvenation. It is noteworthy to mention that human body is a dynamic function and its ability to recover from illnesses is remarkable. Like any other organism, it has a growth pattern that ceases when characteristic size is attained in adulthood. The individual capacity to grow is largely controlled genetically but there are many other factors that interfere with growth mechanism. Lack of specific food constituents can hamper this delicate mechanism, no matter how much dietary carbohydrates and dietary proteins are ingested. Regulated cell growth can not take place unless proper types of lipids are consumed. After adulthood, the compensatory growth mechanism takes over to maintain the gene expression. If this compensatory growth factor is exceeded by necrosis or risk factors, diseases develop. Healthy constitution involves physical as well as neurologic aspects. Thus development of a healthy nervous system becomes an absolute necessity in healing chronic disorders. Neurons like any other cells can be repaired and regenerated. So

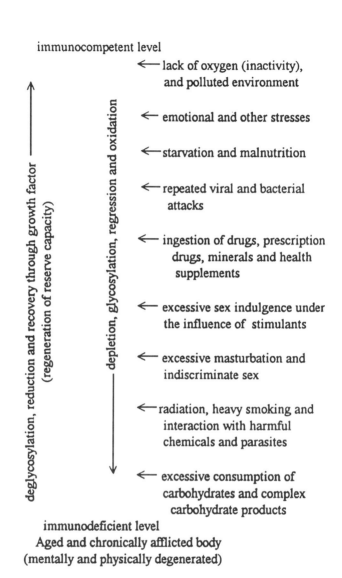

immunocompetent level

← lack of oxygen (inactivity),
and polluted environment

← emotional and other stresses

← starvation and malnutrition

← repeated viral and bacterial
attacks

← ingestion of drugs, prescription
drugs, minerals and health
supplements

← excessive sex indulgence under
the influence of stimulants

← excessive masturbation and
indiscriminate sex

← radiation, heavy smoking and
interaction with harmful
chemicals and parasites

← excessive consumption of
carbohydrates and complex
carbohydrate products

deglycosylation, reduction and recovery through growth factor
(regeneration of reserve capacity)

depletion, glycosylation, regression and oxidation

immunodeficient level
Aged and chronically afflicted body
(mentally and physically degenerated)

Figure 9-1:   Flow chart for restoration process

54

the concept of "Total Healing can be envisioned with growth factor mechanism (Figure 9-1).

©
Kakar Food Classification:

At present there seems to be insufficient knowledge and basic understanding of food constituents and the role they play in pathogenesis and healing. And because conclusively, the answer to total healing lies in the food constituents we consume, I have added this section to introduce my readers to an entirely new concept about food constituents. Based on my experimental work with these materials, I have come to the conclusion that the foods most commonly consumed by humans, fall into three basic classifications. These classifications are based on the principle of relative oxidation potential.

I   Oxidants

      A. Oxygen is the most powerful oxidant and very essential for the reduction-oxidation cycle.

      B.   Carbohydrates:

        * complex carbohydrates such as bleached and unbleached flour

        * corn, potatoes, and grains such as rice, barley, oats and wheat;

        * corn syrup, fructose, sugar and glucose

Glucose is a reductant as compared to oxygen but is a strong oxidant when compared to natural saturated fats and proteins. Body utilizes glucose extensively, as a secondary oxidant when the supply of oxygen is limited. Processing of glucose and its storage in the body as glycogen, requires several enzymes. These enzymes have to be generated by the cells. This is an extra burden for the body to handle such a vast amount of glucose especially when the reserves of healthy lipids are in short supply. This is usually the case with the elderly who have exhausted their healthy lipids and also with individuals who are victims of malignant cancer. It is emphasized that body can live well without complex carbohydrates during healing period. It can produce D- 1,3 diphosphoglyceric acid in situ from lipids, when desired. Since human body tends to consume excessive amount of carbohydrates, it has to pay heavy price in terms of illnesses, premature aging and early death. Carbohydrates are designated here as inflammatory agents.

II. Partially Oxidized Lipids or Partial Reductants

This class includes mono, polyunsaturated and partially hydrogenated vegetable oils such as corn, olive, peanut, soya bean, conola and margarine respectively. They provide protection against many risk factors such as high blood pressure and high cholesterol levels, provided the patient has sufficient amount of healthy subcutaneous fats in the body. Exclusive consumption of these oils over prolonged period, do cause thinning of skin and blood vessels, weight loss, and loss in bone density. They should be avoided during recovery from serious chronic and infectious ailments. For daily consumption these oils should always be mixed with some amount of saturated fats, nuts and green vegetables to counteract their inflammatory characteristics.

56

III. Reductants:

Reductants are classified into two sections: natural fats and proteins. Proteins alone or in combination with lipids generate formidable network of antibodies against inflammatory processes caused by bacteria, parasites and viruses by enhancing various subgrowth factors. They are described here as antioxidants and antiaging compounds. Natural lipids from animal source contain saturated/ unsaturated fats in varying proportion. Saturated fats such as palmitic acid, stearic acid and sphingomyelin are mainly found in the central nervous system. These lipids form plasmic and nuclear membranes of all cells in the body. They also contain cholesterol and its precursor such as squalene from which all steroid hormones are synthesized. They prevent cancer of lymphatic system, epithelial and mucosal linings. These lipids also provide high degree of water repellencey to the cell, thus creating a strong barrier against bacteria and viruses. In lay man's term they are defined as healthy or biofunctional fats. They preserve many organs in the body. They are designated as anti-inflammatory agents.

      A.   Fats in butter, almonds, coconut and coconut milk, nuts, cream and lard or animal fats are quite suitable for daily requirement and are pleasant to consume. Bees wax from honey comb, waxes from hazel nuts, palm nuts, walnuts and spermaceti wax are high molecular weight saturated lipids with unique healing characteristics. The degree of unsaturation is variable but low as compared to monounsaturated oils.

      B.   Proteins found in eggs, seafood, meat (beef, veal, venison and poultry), whole milk and whole milk products such as casein, cheese, yogurt especially from camel and goat milk, legumes, nuts, seeds, and vegetables make essential components of the body. Proteins and amino acids in the body should be protected from oxidation.

Nature has provided us with a variety of products. By selecting proper ratio of reductants to oxidants, one can easily control the growth factor for curing many illnesses. The elderly with lean and fragile bones should eat proteins, animal fat, butter, fruits and vegetables. In order to strengthen the cardiovascular system, they should maintain proper electrolyte balance. In cases such as constipation and heartburn, it is preferable to use magnesium hydroxide in minute concentration. Indiscriminate use of magnesium can adversely affect the central nervous system and cause serious complications in functioning of bones, cartilage, kidneys and muscles.

Oxidants are important for a healthy body to derive energy from cell components but excessive intake should be controlled especially by children during growing period. It is appropriate to consume complex carbohydrates derived from whole grain such as barley, corn, oats and wheat rather than in refined forms. Whole grain may be consumed in boiled, cooked, milled or other suitable form. It has nucleic acid components, essential oils, proteins and free radical quenchers such as vitamin E in addition to complex carbohydrates.

Terms:

Anti-inflammatory   *Antioxidants*
Autonomic nervous system   *Food classification*
Cholesterol   *Sphingomyelin*
Squalene   *Steroid*

10 Healing and Rejuvenation

When healing begins, rejuvenation sets in.
(Kakar)

Age related disorders are reversible provided the damage to the body is not so serious as to be beyond repair. Patients with chronic impairments may be brought back to a healthy condition through specific nutrition, care and exercise. Most of the chronic disorders are caused by prolonged malnutrition or starvation. In chronic or slow starvation which is caused by many factors, cells do not receive enough proteins and lipids for structural and metabolic functions. Before delving into detail, it is noteworthy to mention a few points that pertain to this important subject.

The human body is intimately in tune with nature. Its structural components are unique in their characteristics and have evolved with time. Any alteration in their native structures in the body will have adverse effect on the whole organism. All cellular reactions that take place in the body are tied to the maintenance and reproduction of the organism and collectively to the survival of the cell.

In order to maintain the gene expression such as the human body, an enormous number of series of sequential chemical reactions are needed. For instance, there is an astronomical number of cells in the body and almost every cell contains the exact copy of chromosomes. Realize the amount of DNA constituents needed to make chromosomes and to replace the mutated or damaged segments. All these materials come from fresh food.

Every organ in the human body has a critical mass related to its body weight for peak or optimum performance. When the mass of a particular organ falls below this critical level, lesions develop resulting in the loss of some degree of functionality. Development of a lesion which may be sensed as pain/disease or not, largely depends upon the type of organ involved.

Another point to emphasize is the homeostasis nature of the cell in the body. When there is a sudden change in the microenvironment such as change in concentration of nutrients or accumulation of elements than desired, the cell performance is adversely affected. Absence of oxygen, water, ingestion of alcohol, chemicals, prescription and other drugs or any other unfamiliar agent can abruptly disturb the microenvironment of the cell and in extreme cases cause cell death. Since the treatment described below is related to growth mechanism, it is strongly advised to become involved in moderate activities which stimulate both mind and muscles. Stimulation is the key factor in healing especially while growth is taking place. This can be enhanced when rest is taken after ingesting a meal. Unnecessary emotional and physical stress should be avoided.

©
Methodology

The treatment described in this section may appear simple but it involves fundamental changes in the body chemistry at a molecular level. The reader is advised to consult a physician or a clinical nutritionist with strong medical background who can monitor one's treatment progress on a regular basis before embarking on this project of healing and rejuvenation.

To repair structural, metabolic and molecular damage inflicted by various mechanisms, is an enormous task and requires discipline, patience, understanding, persistent effort on the part of a patient to avoid irritants or agents that harm the body. Every food item mentioned in this treatment has specific significance. A combination of some foods helps the cells to grow and produce enzymes that help digestion and other various metabolic functions and still others have been incorporated to maintain and preserve the cells from over oxidation.

The condition of gastrointestinal tract from buccal cavity to anus determines the status of the nutrients through the digestive tract into the blood. Chronic gastrointestinal disorders such as acidic stomach, constipation, indigestion and stomach ulcer are warning signals for many troubles ahead. They denote that epithelial layers or mucous surfaces throughout the body are under erosion. These eroded mucous linings can not secrete enzymes. This poses a serious problem to the patient as far as food absorption is concerned. These individuals are allergic to many food types and have autoimmune syndrome such as cancer of colon. If the process of erosion is allowed to proceed, other symptoms such as disorders of bones, connective tissues, nervous and respiratory systems may soon appear. Bone ailments such as arthritis, osteoporosis and rheumatoid arthritis are intimately related to immune system.

Thus careful selection of food type becomes mandatory for the sick and aged individuals. The main essence of this therapy is to provide constant supply of dietary saturated fats, nucleic acid components and dietary proteins to replace all the damaged, glycosylated, inflamed or oxidized structures of an organ in the diseased body. For proper cell growth daily intake of food should include eggs, fish, poultry, red meat, beans, lentils, vegetables, fruits and butter. It is advised that ingredients used in cooking should be procured in fresh form and meals should be cooked "at home" under proper supervision. In severe deterioration some percentage of animal fat, coconut milk and coconut may be substituted for butter. In order to optimize the results, the consumption of food ingredients with inflammatory characteristics such as refined carbohydrates and partially oxidized lipids such as margarine, hydrogenated fats, processed vegetable oils ought to be avoided during healing period. Introduction to high protein and moderate amount of natural saturated fats should be done with gradual progression starting with soup containing meat extract, butter and fresh vegetables. Most of the autoimmune ailments are related to rapid metabolism of proteins and lack of healthy adipose tissues. It is emphasized that desired enzymes activity can not take place within the cells without the help of healthy adipose tissues. So dietary proteins and natural saturated fats become the theme of this methodology. It is difficult to suggest a specific protocol to individuals with varied symptoms. All food constituents whether natural saturated fats, carbohydrates or proteins can be harmful to the body if consumed in excessive amount than desired. If some undesirable symptoms such as allergy, mild pain or tightness develop, it may be an indication that there is an imbalance in the consumption of specific food constituents. The logical approach is to check which food constituent is being consumed in excessive amount and which one is left out. It always pays to listen to your body language.

Protocol # 1

This protocol is designed for individuals suffering from autoimmune syndromes. This includes metabolic disorders such as diabetes, hyperthyroidism and pancreatitis; bone and bone marrow disorders such as arthritis, osteoarthritis, osteoporosis; cancer of lymphatic system, mucosal linings and secretive glands; chronic disorders such as chronic fatigue, chronic infection (bacterial, viral and parasitic) and chronic inflammation; defective immune system; neurologic impairments; respiratory infection and skin ailments. This protocol is extremely valuable to individuals suffering from serious immune disorders such as AIDS, leprosy and T.B.

A typical food intake for 150 lbs body may include the following for recuperation on daily basis.

Soup

Prepare meat extract by boiling 1-2 oz of fresh red meat (beef, goat, lamb or pork) till it becomes tender, then add 4oz of fresh green vegetables and 1/4 stick of butter. Initially some individuals whose gastrointestinal tract have become dysfunctional may react unfavorably to this protocol. After adjusting to above food intake, the following may be tried three to four times a week for a brief period under physician guidance. For patients with serious illnesses this protocol should be followed on daily basis.

Breakfast:

        1-2 eggs (scrambled or in any other form in butter)
        1 to 3 oz fresh meat (beef, goat, lamb or pork)
        4 oz fresh steamed green vegetables in butter
        1 glass of fruit juice

Lunch:

        2-4 oz fresh leafy vegetables or salad with
            sardines
        1   cup of yogurt or milk
        1   fruit of any kind (in case of stomach
            disorders avoid oranges)

Dinner:

        2-3 oz of cooked vegetables in butter
        1   cup of lentil or bean soup fried in butter
        2-3 oz rice (can be substituted with potatoes,
            sweet corn, whole grain flour)

Since we are dealing with growth process, proper electrolyte balance is essential to achieve desired results. Excess of one electrolyte over another can cause serious complications or even death . The daily intake of butter is left to individual. Normal fat requirement varies depending on the severity of the condition. It is suggested not to consume any other lipids than natural saturated fats during healing period. The snacks in between meals should include roasted peanuts, nuts, cheese, dried fish and naturally occurring proteins items with fats. Unlimited variations of above recipes can be designed to suit your taste by using slight imagination. At least one meal should be without carbohydrates such as wheat, flour, pasta, potatoes and rice. Morning meals should include proteins and natural fats to generate enzymes that are needed to produce structural components. The amount of fats can be varied from 5- 30% depending upon the ability of the patient to digest fats. This will cause changes in the concentration of proteins. Excessive consumption of meat over a long period, can cause serious complications such as contraction of blood vessels and ischemia of heart muscles. Most of the heart attacks in healthy individuals are caused by excessive accumulation of iron in the body. If such a situation arises, it can be resolved by discontinuing its consumption for a brief period. Treat your food as the ultimate medicine and use analysis and judgment before you sit for a meal. The distinct feature of the above protocol is that it has all the elements for making collagen such as amino acids, vitamin C and iron except molecular oxygen. Lack of oxygen as well as any of these components can lead to abnormal collagen that can not form fibers. Malfunction in collagen formation or alteration in collagen structure results in fragile blood vessels and lesions in many organs. The status of collagen is intertwined with cell characteristics. They go hand in hand as distinct unit to form various organs in the body. Individuals who work in closed environment are likely to develop infection and degenerative disorders as compared to their counterparts who work in open air. Inactivity over a long period of time does result in the degeneration of bones, muscles and nerves even in individuals who consume right kind of food constituents. People who lead sedentary life lose collagen very rapidly and develop cardiovascular disorders due to rapid loss in cell density.

Protocol #2

This protocol may be substituted for protocol #1 and is designed for individuals who dislike red meat. This could be due to religious reasons or aversion developed by high levels of iron in the body.

Breakfast:

> 1-2 eggs fried in butter
> 4 oz steamed or broiled fish in butter
> 2 oz steamed vegetables in butter
> 1 cup freshly squeezed fruit juice

For lunch and dinner follow protocol #1. Some individuals who are allergic to sea food may try fowls such as chicken or duck.

Protocol #3

This protocol is designed exclusively for vegetarians. It could also be used for individuals who have developed other disorders as mentioned in protocol #1 in addition to cardiovascular ailments. It has been found to be useful for patients with neuromuscular, neurovascular and musculoskeletal disorders. The good source of proteins are moong, chick peas, beans, lentils and milk products. Nuts of all kinds including almonds, coconut, palm nuts and roasted pea nuts are excellent source of not only proteins but also vitamin B complex, calcium, iron, magnesium, zinc and natural fats. Vegetarian have to rely heavily on whole milk, milk products for healthy proteins and fats such as butter and cream which include vitamins such as A, B

66

complex, D and E.

©
Effect of magnesium in rejuvenation:

Magnesium is a unique mineral in healing many debilitating disorders. It is the basic mineral that is essential for genetic machinery and helps in the growth mechanism. Magnesium is extremely useful in relaxing muscles and preventing high blood pressure and many other cardiovascular disorders. It is also responsible for for making high density lipoproteins which reduce coronary heart disease. Magnesium role as a cofactor in many enzymatic reactions is well known. It is essential to normal functioning of bones, musclesnerves and gene replication. It also plays an important part in making supramolecular structures of many organs of the body. Magnesium is usually found in grains, legumes, fruits, vegetables and milk. It has been found that people who drink soft water have higher incidence of developing heart disease than those who are supplied with hard water. The obvious reason is the presence of magnesium in hard water. The daily requirement of total magnesium is 1300 mg per day. This amount should be exclusively derived from natural products such as fruits, nuts, milk and vegetables.

Electrolyte Balance:

Electrolytes play crucial role in regulation and coordination of muscular as well as neuromuscular activities. Sudden changes in their concentration can cause complications and in extreme cases death. It is very difficult to maintain electrolyte balance in an unhealthy tissue or an organ. But there is immediate need of electrolytes such as potassium, magnesium, calcium, zinc and iron during the growth of healthy organs and organ systems. Magnesium and potassium deficiency exists among the elderly population who consume alcohol, meat, calcium, iron supplements and prescription drugs. During recovery from chronic illnesses, restricted amount of magnesium may be needed to generate bones, muscles and nerves. Hypomagnesinimia can develop in conditions such as malabsorption, surgery, malnutrition and alcoholism, which can result in symptoms such as mental confusion, muscle weakness, stiffness and poor muscle co-ordination. As iron is essential for collagen synthesis, so is magnesium for relaxation of muscles of blood vessels, eyes, heart and legs. My own investigation has shown that certain correlation exists between iron, calcium, magnesium, potassium and sodium. Iron and calcium can replace potassium and magnesium and magnesium can displace iron as well as calcium in the body. Excessive use of magnesium is not recommended because it can cause ischemia of muscles due to loss of potassium and calcium and can cause severe damage to the nervous system. Proper intake of minerals such as calcium, magnesium, sodium, potassium in form of juices, milk, fruits and vegetables, becomes extremely important during such therapy. It is emphasized that no single food item ingested can bring forth desired results. In order to achieve optimum results all the ingredients must be consumed on daily basis.

©

Kakar Period of Reduction or Deglycosylation:

As described previously that an aged or diseased body is either depleted or glycosylated, in other words oxidized like rusted iron. Before any significant improvement can be seen in the patient, the glycosylated protein structures have to be

68

deglycosylated which is achieved through generating new enzymes. In order to make highly effective enzymes, it is suggested that consumption of simple and complex carbohydrates should be reduced to minimal amount during healing period. Recovery period depends upon the extent of glycosylation or oxidation, exposure to irritants, absorption of nutrients and availability of fresh air and water. This recovery period is hereby defined as Kakar Period of Deglycosylation, which is defined as the time required to deglycosylate the afflicted body to a desired level of glycosylation.

In this therapy consumption of liquor, smoking, drugs (chemical agents, narcotics, prescription drugs which harm the cells), hot spices, vitamins and mineral supplements are not recommended. Moderate exercise is essential to supply nutrients and oxygen to every part of the body. A word of caution pertaining to exercise is advised for individuals who are ridden with arthritis and osteoporosis. The body will automatically give signals to engage in exercise. Stiff muscles and bones will show flexibility after sometimes due to regulated cell growth. By this technique bones and muscle mass may be increased and many bone deformities may be alleviated by following this therapy. Behavioral disorders such as depression, mood swings, phobias and other disorders related to central nervous system may be healed. This therapy is extremely useful to victims of AIDS, leprosy, T.B., fire and radiation burns. In reality, any human disorder can be healed by this technique. *This methodology may not be beneficial to those who have bone spurs, gallstones, kidney stone or some kind of obstruction in heart and blood vessels. These acute cases may require immediate medical attention. However, after the operation, further erosion may be brought under control by using this unique technique.

It is imperative to mention about other techniques that may be found to be equally effective, in reducing the oxidation potential of inflamed or infected tissues *in situ* such as blood, genes, enzymes, antibodies, tumors lesions, etc. are;

(i) treatment of blood (antigens), lymphatic fluid (antibodies) and organs with steady stream of protons generated by various methods and

(ii) treatment of affected tissues or body with lipids and proteins, high density lipoproteins, nucleoproteins, lipo-nucleoproteins and hydrolysed derivatives obtained from various tissues and organs of animals and plants by various routes.

These methods may shrink soft tumors, change markers on antibodies, red blood cells and tissues, and boost the immune system for a brief period. But for severe chronic illnesses, it is preferable to use precursors such natural lipids, proteins, nucleic acid components, minerals and vitamins in dietary form, to generate healthy subgrowth factors of various types, to repair the damaged tissues.

Terms:

Buccal cavity	Hyrolysed	Markers
Cofactor	Hypercalcemia	Membranes
Gene expression	Kidney stone	Precursors
Gallstone	Lymphatic	Protons
Antigen-antibody		Hypomagnesinimia

The following disorders can be effectively cured provided the damage to the tissues, organs or body is not extensive.

Age related disorders;

random deterioration or aging hits, decline in organ functions and anatomical modifications, maturity onset diabetes, glaucoma, dim vision and premature cataractogenesis.

Bone disorders;

abnormalities in bone marrow and bone mass production, arthritis, back pains, osteoporosis, osteoarthritis and rheumatoid arthritis.

Cardiovascular disorders;

abnormalities caused by erosion of endothelial layers, or due to degeneration of collagen and connective tissues of blood vessels

Carcinogenesis;

cancer of bladder, brain, breast, connective tissues, liver, mucous membranes, liver, lymph nodes, ovary, pancreas, prostate, salivary glands, skin and vagina

Gastrointestinal disorders:	acidic stomach, peptic ulcerative colitis, and malabsorption.
General chronic disorders:	anorexia nervosa, chronic fatigue, chronic infection and chronic inflammation.
Immune system:	hypersensitivity and autoimmune syndrome such as chronic infection, leprosy, T.B. and AIDS.
Metabolic disorders:	diabetes, pancreatitis, hypo and hyper insulinism, hyperparathyroidism and dysfunction of endocrine secretions such as hormones
Nervous disorders;	depression, nervousness, phobias, multiple sclerosis, epilepsy, paralysis and erosion of epithelial linings in brains.
Respiratory disorders;	common cold, chronic bronchitis, hay fever and sinusitis
Skin disorders;	chronic itching, fungal infection, parakeratosis, psoriasis, loss of hair, pigment and skin cancers.

11   Conclusion and Perspectives

All information on genes are kept in the reduced form.
                                                          (Kakar)

In summing up it is suffice to say that a healthy state is a dynamic state when the forces of disintegration are exceeded by the forces generated by cell synthesis and cell-cell interaction and any deviation from this state of health is defined as illness. The degenerative forces are emotional and physical stress, pressure, radiation, temperature, harmful chemical agents, drugs, bacteria, viruses, malnutrition and starvation.

In all of my discussion, I have clearly spelled out cell as a unit in which DNA is complexed with proteins, RNA including organelles surrounded by membranes. There are two distinct processes that are taking place; one is the process of synthesis, DNA$\rightarrow$ RNA$\rightarrow$ proteins and the other is the process of oxidation. In order to make the genetic apparatus perform with great fidelity, it has to be protected from the forces of oxidation and disintegration. One can easily realize the importance of membranes that surround the nucleus and the organelles. The genetic apparatus is utterly dysfunctional without them. Its functionality as a useful entity heavily rests upon the types of lipids consumed for making cells. Natural saturated fats provide maximum protection as compared to unsaturated fats against the harsh environment in which we live. The latter have the tendency to undergo oxidation especially when they are stripped off of free radical quenchers. Oxidation processes grossly distort the shapes of the cells.

Diffusion of oxygen through these lesions can cause cascade type of deterioration starting from the enzymes of the plasmic membrane leading to regulatory proteins and DNA.

It is emphasized that oxidation can not take place unless there is a corresponding reductant to release electrons. The higher the intensity of reduction potential, the higher the efficiency of cells to produce enzymes, immunoglobulins and specific proteins for many organs of the body. So constant supply of reductants becomes essential for the health of cells. Many neurologic impairments such as Alzheimer's disease, confused brain syndrome, depression, neurosis, multiple sclerosis and phobias are caused by degeneration of nerve cells.

The genetic machinery that we inherit in the form of fertilized egg seems perpetual. The most distinct feature of this unique machinery is the replication process which goes on and on with extreme rapidity. This process is quite universal and makes the growth process possible in all living things. Gene expression can not take place unless genes interact with constituents such as fats, proteins, nucleic acids and carbohydrates. The ratio in which these constituents interact with genetic machinery and the manner in which they react with one another, can have profound effect on gene expression. Since gene expression takes place incessantly, continual supply of food constituents becomes of prime importance. It is an admitted fact that gene expression will be defective if we do not feed our body with right constituents or merely feed it with prescription drugs or chemicals that destroy cell components and cell metabolism. Healthy body has healthy genes expression and vice versa. Since gene expression is a delicate process and sensitive to many risk factors (in lay man's term means stress), it is logical to avoid foods that are adulterated, altered, extracted, fermented, infected, modified, radiated reconstituted, separated, synthesized, tainted, bleached, brominated and oxidized. It is advised not to ingest antacid pills, minerals supplements and other health derivatives. These materials may seem innocuous and in some cases may show positive outcome for a brief period, but in the long run their effects are devastating on immune system and neuromuscular network.

Growth factor which involves cellular growth, morphogenesis and cellular differentiation, is the most powerful and unique phenomenon of nature. It is a mechanism through which biological monomers continuously organize themselves into intricate, highly organized entity called organism that can express emotions, perform formidable tasks, think, analyze, perceive and can interact with its environment. An individual during his life time, may generate growth factor of various oxidation potentials, depending upon the lifestyle he maintains and types of food constituents he ingests.

The growth factor of high reduction potential may be used not only to repair/revive mutated genes but to heal lesions, to grow bones, healthy bone marrow, breast, muscles, nerves and hair and replace the damaged tissues from blood vessels, eyes, ears, skin and many other internal parts of the body. It may heal any pathological disorder confronting humans and if properly maintained may delay or even reverse the process of aging. This may bring vigor, vitality and happiness even in advanced stage of life;

In final statement it is concluded that human body is designed to be ageless and works on the same principle as rocket except for the fact the former makes its own hardwares and moves at a slower pace. The longevity of a living organism solely depends upon how it maintains its growth and redox mechanisms and protects itself from environmental hazards. .

Index

Lipoproteoglycans 27
Lubricants 22
Lymphoid organs 48
Lymphocytes 48
Lymph nodes 16
Lysosomes 10

Macromolecules 40
Macrophages 31,48
Magnesium 58,64,67
Magnesium channels 46
Malnutrition 13
Margarine 56
Mathematical model 32
Melanocytes 39
Membranes 8
Metastasize 49
Methodology 60
Minerals 23,67,68
Mystifying molecules 20
Mitochondria 8
Molecular diseases 10
Monocytes 47
Mono unsaturated fats 56
Morbid obesity 50
Mumps 12
Musculoskeletal system 45
Multiple sclerosis 44
Mutated segments 60
Mutation 32
Myasthenia gravis 46
Myelin sheath 45
Myoblasts 39
Myosin 46

NADH 18
Natural saturated
    fats 19,29,33,57,42
Necrosis factors 36,37
Neoplasia 23
Neuroblasts 39
Neurons 45
Neuromuscular
    junctions 46
Neuromuscular
    transmission 46
Neutrophils 48
Nitrogen 4
Nobel gases 4
Nucleic acid 5,8,18,34
Nucleotides 38
Nutrients 13

Oats 55
OK recovery factor 32,33
Optimum yield 24
Organic matrix 45
Organelles 8, 30
Osteoarthritis 63
Osteoporosis 28,63
Output 39
Oxidants 20,55
Oxidative phosphorylation 40
Oxidative burst 10

Palpitation 43
Pancreas 49
Papilloma 11
Parkinson's disease 44

Paramagnetic 17
Pathogens 12
Peanut 64
Peroxy radical 11
Phagocytic activity 48
Phobias 44,72
Phospholipids 8
Photolysis 5
Photosynthesis 4
Plasma cells 47
Polluted environment 54
Polyanions 16
Polymeric materials 2
Polymyositis 46
Polyunsaturated oils 56
Prostate 49
Proteoglycans 16,27
Proteolipids 27
Protozoa 11
Psychosomatic 10
Pumps 22

Ribonucleic acid 8
    (RNA)
Radiation 11,17
Reductants 21,57
Reductases 24
Reduction-oxidation
        potential 18,33
Regulated cell growth 23
Regulatory proteins 30
Relative oxidation 55
Rejuvenation 59
Rheumatoid arthritis 28,46,61

Schiff's base 17
Senility 44
Sensitized cells 48
Soybean oil 56
Squamous cells 11
Stearic acid 20
Stem cells 39
Stiffness 30
Sugar moieties 23
Supressor cells 48
Supramolecular
    structures 58

T-cells 48
Three component
        model 26
Thymus 49
Total healing 52
Toxin 10
Transducer 32
Tricarboxylic
    acid cycle 18
Triglycerides 6
Tumor 40

UV radiation 11
Ulcer 61
Unbleached flour 55
Unmyelinated axons 45
Uremia 40
    Visual disorders 45
Vitamins 11

FURTHER READING:

1- Arms, K. and Camp, P.S.; Biology, 2nd. Ed., Saunder College Publishing, 1982.

2- Bettelheim, F.A. and Kakar, S.K.; Hydration of Actin, Invet. Opthalmol. Vis, 32, 562-564,1991.

3- Boyd, W. and Sheldon, H.; Introduction to the study of diseases, 8th Ed., Philadelphia, Lea and Febiger, 1980.

4- Bourne, G.H.; Biochemistry and Physiology of bones, vol.I, II and III, 2nd Ed., Academic Press, 1972.

5- Budy, A. M.; Biology of Hard Tissue, Proceedings of second conference, National Aeronautics and Space Administration, 1968.

6- Bullough, W.S.; Epidermal, epidermal mitosis in relation to sugar and phosphate, Nature, Vol. 163, 660, 1949.

7- Crocco, J.A.; Gray's Anatomy, A revised american from the fifteenth English Edition, 1977.

8- De Roberts, E.D. Nowinski, W.W.; Saez, F.A., Cell Biology, 4th Ed., W.A. Saunders, 1965.

9- Frost, H.M.; The physiology of Cartilaginous Fibrous and Bony Tissue, Springfield, Ill., Charles C. Thomas Publisher, 1972.

10- Hawkes, S. and Wang, J.L.; Extra Cellular Matrix, Academic Press, 1982.

11- Hay, E.D.; Cell- matrix interaction in Embrynoic avian cornea and lens in Extra Cellular Matrix by Hawkes, S. and Wang, J.L., Academic press, 1982.

12- Heino, J. et al; Regulation of cell adhesion by transforming growth factor beta, co-comitant regulation of the integrin that store beta sub unit, J. Bio. Chem. 264, 380, 1989.

13- Hyda, K.K. et al.; Interaction and assembly of basement membrane and components in Extra Cellular Matrix by Hawkes, S. and Wang, J. L., Academic Press, 1982

14- Ignotz, R.A. et al.; Regulation of cell adhesion receptors by transforming growth factor beta regulation of vitronection receptor and LFA-1, J. Bio., 264, 389, 1989.

15- Kirk, D. L.; Biology Today, Random House Inc., 1980.

16- Kupper, T.S.; Immune and Inflammatory processes in cutaneous tissues, J. Clin. Invest., 86, 1783-1789, 1990.

17- Kanungo, M.S.; Biochemistry of Aging, Academic Press, 1980.

18- Mazur, A. and Harrow, B.; Text Book of Biochemistry, 10th Ed., W. B. Saunders Company, 1971.

19- Metzler, D.E.; Biochemistry, The chemical reaction of the living cell, Academic Press, 1977.

20- Miller, F.N.; Peery and Miller's Pathology, 3rd Ed., Academic Press, 1978.

21- Montagana, W.; The structure and Function of Skin, 2nd Ed., Academic Press, 1975.

22- Neal, A.L.; Chemistry and Biochemistry, a comprehensive introduction, McGraw-Hill, 1971.

23- Neurath, H. and Bailey, K.; Proteins, Vol. 1, Part B. Academic Press, 1953.

24- Neurath, H., Hill. R.L. and Boeder, C.L.; Proteins, 3rd Ed., Vol.1, Academic Press, 1975.

25 Nicklooff et al.; American Journal of Pathol., 138, 129, 1991.

26- Parrish, J.A.; Dematology and Skin Care, McGraw-Hill Company, 1973.

27- Peter Banks, J. of NIH, 1, 93, 1989.

28- Purandare, Y.K.; Lecture Notes on Physiologycal Chemistry, 1987.

29- Rennine, J.; The body against itself, Scientific American, 263, #6, 106, 1990.

30- Ruoslashti, E. and Pierschbacher, New prospectives in cell adhesion; RG Integrins, Science, 239, 491, 1987.

31- Russel, P.J.; Genetics, 2nd Ed., Scoot, Foresman and Co., 1988.

32- Shipman, P., Walker, A. and Bichell, D., The Human Skeleton, Harvard University Press, 1985.

33- Smith, K.A.; Interleukin-2; Scientific American, 262, 50, 1990.

34- Spetor, R. and Johonson, C.E.; The mammalian choroid plexus, Scientific American, Vol.261, #5,1989.

35- Sutton, R. and Waisman,M.; The Practitioner' Dermatology, 1st Ed., Dun-Donelley Publishing Corporation, 1973.

36- Szilard,L.; Nature, 184, 958-960, 1959.

37- Trump, B.F. and Arstilla, A.U.; Cellular reaction to injury by Lavia, M.F. and Hill, Jr. R.B., 2nd Ed., Oxford University Press, 1975.

38- Vander, A.J., Sherman, J.H. and Luciano, D.S., Human Physiology, the mechanism of body function, McGraw -Hill Inc., 1980.

39- Villee, C.A., Solomon, E.P. and Davis, P.W.; Biology, Saunder College Publishing, 1985.

40- Waston, J.D.; Molecular Biology of the Gene, Menlow Park, Calif., Benjamin-Cummings, 1976.

GLOSSARY

Acetylcholine- acetic acid derivative of choline; the neurotransmitter
    used by cholinergic nerves.

Actin- a muscle fiber which in conjunction with mysosin is responsible
    for the ability of muscles to contract; actin and myosin are
    protein components of the muscle fibers.

Adaptive immunity - immunity achieved by generating antibodies
    against a particular antigen by the body.

Adenosine triphosphate (ATP)- an important substance used in
    transferring energy from biochemical reactions that give up
    energy to those that need it.

Adipose tissue- a type of connective tissue containing fat cells.

AIDS- Acquired Immunity Deficiency Syndrome.

Allergy- hypersensitivity of an individual to a substance in amount
    harmless to others; adverse reaction is reflected by changes
    in various body tissues.

Alzheimer' disease- neurofibrillary degeneration. Senile plaques are
    seen in gray cortex. The symptoms are those of senile
    dementia such as forgetfulness followed by irritability
    and the irrationality.

Anaphylaxis- type-1 (hay-fever)- symptoms include nasal congestion,
    sneezing, running nose and itching of the eyes. In Type II the
    antigen binds to red and white blood cells or platelets. In type
    III antigen-antibody complex is deposited on the walls of
    blood vessels. Type IV (delayed hypersensitivity) is
    encountered in contact dermatitis and poison ivy.

Antiaging compounds- substances that prevent aging processes in the body.

Antibody- immunoglobulins produced by plasma cells in response to specific antigen and have the capacity to react against bacteria, viruses and toxins.

Antigen- foreign substance which, if introduced into the body may lead to antibody formation. Bacteria, viruses, proteins and toxins may act as antigen.

Antioxidant- substance that prevents the oxidation processes in the body. This definition differs from the common terminology used for antioxidants by health industry.

Arachnoid membrane- the middle of the three meningeal layers.

Autoimmune syndrome (body against itself); individual may develop antibodies to a substance formed in his own body.

Autonomic nervous system- that portion of the nervous system that regulates muscles and glands thereby helping to maintain homeostasis

Axon- long tubular portion of the neuron cell body.

Bone marrow disorders- types of leukemia; lymphogenous and myelogenous.

Buccal cavity- portion pertaining to mouth.

Chondrontine sulfate- a substance of basement membrane

Chromosomal aberration- defect or mutation in which large segment of chromosomes are deleted, duplicated or transloacted.

Collagen- a primary protein component of tendons, ligaments, skin, bone and cartilage.

Concentration flux or gradient- forward flow or movement of enzymes, immunoglobulins and structural proteins etc.

Cytotoxic T cell- T cells that kill antigenic cells directly.

Delayed hypersensitivity- Anaphylaxis type IV is mediated by T lymphocytes. The reaction takes twelve hours to develop. Posion ivy, contact dermatitis and eczema are examples of this type of allergy.

Deoxyribose- a reduced ribose sugar molecule.

Depurination- the breakdown of purine molecule.

Deoxyribonucleic acid (DNA) replication- the formation of exact copy of DNA segment.

Dysplasia- the abnormal development of a tissue

Electrochemical potential barrier- barrier created by hydrogen atoms bearing molecules.

Electron transport - the transfer of electrons from one system to another.

Entropy- a measure of the extent of disorder in a system.

Enzyme- a protein molecule that acts as catalyst to promote or regulate biochemical reaction/s.

Epithelial tissue or epithelium- continuous layer or sheet covering the body surface or lining of a cavity. These layers consist of cells fitted tightly together.

Extracellular matrix- relates to basement membrane or the layer that lies below the basal surface of epithelium such as skin. It contains collagen, heparan sulfate, laminin and enactin.

FADH- hydrogen bound form of flavin adenine dinucleotides or FAD as a hydrogen carrier.

Food classification- This term was coined by the author based on his experimental studies. Foods can be conveniently categorized into oxidants, partially oxidized components and reductants based on relative redox potential. Oxidants (inflammatory) such as carbohydrates and many sugar derivatives are needed in the body to conduct catabolic activities in the body or used to balance the excessive effect of reductants to generate energy in the body. Reductants (anti-inflammatory) or risk reducing food constituents such as fats and proteins, are essential for the body to make new cells and enzymes thereby resisting the effect of necrosis or risk factors such as carbohydrates, bacteria, viruses, chemical agents, temperature and pressure.

Growth factor- the rate of protein synthesis which involves the interaction of dietary fats and proteins with genes. Many risk factors undermine this growth factor which leads to pathogenesis (disease formation). Forward flux of growth factor is a sort of replacement technique to replace the old or damaged cells by the new ones, from the body.

Gene expression- the development of an organism from inherited genes.

Genetic machinery- the inherited genes such as fertilized egg.

Genetic mutation- any inherited change in the sequence of DNA.

Glycosaminoglycans- a substance of extracellular matrix or basement membrane.

Glycosylated lipids- a substance formed from lipids or fats and glucose; glycosylated lipoprotein - product formed from glucose, proteins and lipids interaction; glycosylated nucleic acid are formed from nucleic acid and glucose.

Heparan sulfate- a substance of extracellular matrix.

Heparin- a substance of basement membrane.

Homeostasis- the balanced internal environment such as temperature etc..

Humoral response- the production of antibodies by plasma cells located on the lymph nodes whereas in the cell mediated response, T cells travel to the invasion site.

Hydroxy radical- radical formed in free radical mechanism.

Hyaluronic acid- a component of the basement membrane.

Hydrolases- enzymes that conducts the process of hydrolysis.

Hyperglycemia (glycosuria) - in a condition where glucose in blood is elevated. This could be due to insufficient production of insulin; hypoinsulinism otherwise known diabetes mellitus.

Hyperplasia- the increase in number of cells.

Hypoglycemia- in a condition where glucose level in the blood is abnormally low; hyperinsulinism is caused by the presence of a tumor.

Immunoglobulins- antibodies formed in response to specific antigen.

Inflammation- characterized by redness, pain and swelling; caused by many risk factors.

Keratan sulfate- a component of basement membrane.

Kreb's cycle- the final common pathway for the oxidation of pyruvic acid, fatty acids and the carbon chains of amino acids.

Ligaments- strong connecting band of tough, flexible, fibrous
   tissues joining two bones

Lymphoid- pertaining to cellular structure similar to the tissue
   of lymph glands.

Lymphocytes- white blood cells.

Lysosomes - a cytoplasmic organelle containing digestive enzymes.

Macromolecules- large molecules, a term applied to polymers.

Macrophages- cells that engulf microorganisms and foreign matter.

Melanocytes- pigment forming cells.

Metastasize- the transfer of a disease from one part of the body to
   another.

Mitochondria- cellular organelles that are the sites of cellular
   respiration.

Molecular disease- presence of disease at molecular level.

Musculoskeletal system- pertaining to muscles and bones.

Myasthenia gravis- disease of muscles.

Myelin sheath- the fatty insulating covering around the axons
   of neurons.

Myoblast- muscle forming cells.

NADH- hydrogen bound form of nicotine amide adenine
   dinucleotides.

Necrosis factors- risk factors or factors that tend to destroy cells.

Neoplasia- new growth, term applied to benign and
    malignant tumors.
Neuroblast- neuron forming cells.

Organelle- a specialized functional part of the cell.

Oxidative phosphorylation- the flow of electrons coupled
    to phosphorylation process.

Papilloma- a small nodule of duct of epithelium covering
    a fibrovascular core.

Paramagnetic- substances that become weakly mangetized
    when placed in magnetic field.

Plasma cells- secrete antibodies; differentiated B lymphocytes.

Polyanions- ploymers containing negative charges such as
    polycarboxylic acid.

Polymyositis - a systemic disorder of connective tissue that
    results in inflammatory and degenerative changes in
    voluntary muscles.

Ribonucleic acid (RNA)- functions in the expression of cell's
    genetic information.

Reductants- compounds that prevent the oxidation of cell
    components and reduce the effect of risk factors.
    Saturated fats are classical examples.

Schiff's base- product formed from the interaction of amino
    group with aldehyde.

Squamous cells- flat and scale like cells

Unmyelinated axons- condition in which the myelin sheath
    on the axons of neurons are destroyed.

Nota Bene:

The methodology described in this book may appear simple but involves fundamental changes in the body chemistry of the patient. This approach may not be beneficial to those individuals who have bone spurs, gallstones, kidney stones or some kind of obstruction in flow mechanism in any part of the body. No self - medication/cure is being prescribed and where necessary, seek proper medical advice. Some of the prescription drugs may react adversely with this type methodology because of the sensitive nature of the newly generated cells.

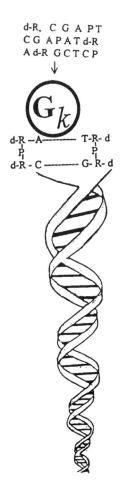

PLATE -II: This diagram depicts the continuous formation of new generation of healthy genes from raw materials. Deleted, mutated or segments with lesions can be repaired/replaced by using the growth factor technique.

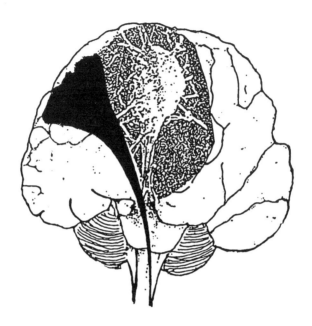

PLATE - III: The diagram shows the healing of demyelinated sheath.
It also shows the development of connective tissues of
cerebral cortex and other neuro-musculovascular network.
Healthy neural network which includes spinal column and
rest of the body, can be grown by using the technique of
forward flux of growth factor.

About the author

Sharwan Kumar Kakar received his B.Sc. (Hons.) in chemistry from Delhi University; B.Sc.(Tech.) in textile chemistry from the Department of Chemical Technology, Bombay University, India; M.S. in textile chemistry from N.C. State University, Raleigh, N.C., U.S.A., and Ph.D. in textile chemistry from Leeds University, Leeds, U.K. He worked as Post Doctoral Fellow on cataractogenesis and muscle fibers under N.I.H. grant, at Adelphi University, Garden City, N.Y. U.S.A.. Dr. Kakar is a life long researcher and has many publications in the field of analytical chemistry, biopolymer science, organic chemistry, polymer science, and textile chemistry. He worked in several organizations as a senior researcher in the field of applied chemistry. He is pioneer in the field of "GROWTH FACTOR" and established the unique concept of "Forward Flux of Growth Factor". He is currently teaching health science courses as an adjunct professor in chemistry department at S.U.N.Y, College of Technology, Farmingdale, and Nassau Community College, Garden City, L.I., N.Y..